THE BEST DECISION
WE EVER MADE

Inspired and created by
VANESSA A. MCDONALD

To Nate Bihlmaier… "Make no small plans."
You are missed, my friend.

CONTENTS

INTRODUCTION

I never intended to write a book. But as the universe placed signs in my life, on my path—I couldn't deny them. I proceeded to follow my intuition, and here we are with *The Best Decision We Ever Made*. Thank you for picking it up to read, or maybe it was given to you. Either way, I hope something in here resonates with you and inspires you to be more curious about your relationship with alcohol.

When I contemplated getting sober, I wrestled with so many questions. Even the word *sober* sounds like *somber*, which often means sad and quiet or too serious. That wasn't very appealing. For some reason, I felt I had to label myself as an alcoholic to stop drinking. I didn't know the exact definition and was reluctant to research to find out. Whether I was an alcoholic or not, I knew drinking was not doing me any favors, and it had to go.

I had no idea how to start—alcohol seemed to be everywhere in my life, and it was becoming easier to access. How would I relax after a long day of work? How would I properly celebrate a big work win? How would I numb the big feelings that sometimes overwhelmed me? How would I go on a vacation without drinking? It seemed all too much, so I continued to drink.

When I thought about where I could get help (I didn't know anyone sober to whom I could open up), all I knew was Alcoholics

Anonymous, and from what I had heard, it didn't sound like a fun place to go. Besides, what if someone saw me there? Someone I knew or who knew my parents? That sounded like a horrible, scary idea.

And I still didn't even know if I was an alcoholic. I had never done anything in order in my life—how could I do 12 steps in a row? What if I failed? What if I drank again? How would that make me feel? I contemplated rehab, but I didn't want to be away from my children for that long.

Right after I stopped drinking, on March 16, 2020, I found TLC—The Luckiest Club. This online, modern recovery community gave me the life I was supposed to have. This community of amazing humans loved me when I couldn't love myself and guided me through forgiveness, redemption, and ultimately freedom. They helped me get past the regret, shame, and embarrassment that comes from drinking too much over 24-plus years. The wisdom that came from the members of this group accelerated my journey, and I wouldn't be here without them.

I'm forever grateful that many of my new friends agreed to contribute to this book. It's an absolute honor to share their insights, experiences, trials, and tribulations with you.

For this book, I compiled a list of questions I wish I could have asked someone before I got sober. Each contributor agreed to answer one of these questions, and their stories appear in no particular order:

- Which is more challenging: the early days of quitting drinking or *staying* alcohol-free? What makes it harder?
- What have you done on a regular basis to help keep you sober?
- What has surprised you most about living an alcohol-free life?
- What advice would you give your Day 1 self?
- How have your daily patterns, relationships, and energy changed?

- What didn't you know about the effects of alcohol on your body and brain?
- In what ways did you deny you had an issue with drinking?
- What held you back from living an alcohol-free life?
- Did your "rock bottom" dictate your decision to get sober, or in what other way did your Day 1 find you?

I hope that through the answers to these questions, you find yourself more open to removing alcohol from your life. If you're wondering if it's worth it, I'll share a simple fact with you: I've looked, and I can't find one person who regrets getting sober.

A.F.S.

Self-proclaimed retired party girl. Self-proclaimed "boring without booze." Sober since March of 2020. Self-proclaimed way more interesting without booze. Loud laughter.

I stay sober by being aware of myself and not staying silent in my struggle. I never shared my problem with alcohol with anyone, and that is precisely what kept me in it for so long.

Shame exists because it festers within us when we are alone and try to hide it. When we begin to speak about it, it begins to lose its power over us. So, now, that is what I do. I speak about it. I use my people—friends and family who love and support me— to help me when I notice I am slipping low. I tell my few that I keep close when I feel vulnerable.

I have become increasingly aware of feelings that make me uncomfortable and how my natural tendency is to numb them away—to drink them away. Now, I do not numb them, but I force myself to get curious about them. I frequently ask myself what I am feeling and have learned to identify those feelings. When I can identify them, I can begin to understand them.

The more I understand myself, the less I judge myself. The less I judge myself, the more I like myself. I did not like myself when I was drinking because I didn't understand who I was or why I did the things I did. When we learn about ourselves, we can begin to practice self-compassion for our past selves. Then we lose the need to numb away the pain. I talk about all of this with people I love and feel safe with. In moments when I am feeling shameful—because those moments still happen—instead of getting quiet and isolating myself, I tell my people that I am noticing feelings of shame coming up. I tell them when a drink sounds good, or I am feeling lonely, or I am driving past bars more often than I need to. I tell them when I have a day exuding of gratitude, and I tell them when my day was full of self-pity. I tell them when it is a combination of the two. I tell them when I'm angry, jealous, sad, and disappointed. I also tell them when I am happy, excited, grateful and calm. Most times, we don't even need to go through the entire processing of what we're experiencing cognitively and emotionally; simply sharing our thoughts and fears with another person lightens the load. The more we share, the more we stay in the light. I always want to be in the light, now. It does not feel as heavy as the dark.

Struggling alone is what keeps us in the dark for so long. If you can find just one person to stay in the light with, it is enough. You just need one. Having one person that you can text to, vent to, be honest with, tell them about how great or horrible of a day you had, is really all you need. One person with whom you can be truly authentic is enough to change the course of your sobriety. When we allow ourselves to finally speak and get vulnerable about our struggles, we can be free to be ourselves.

Despite what the shame spiral of booze told us, being ourselves is the best place to be, really. It is freeing, and we cannot have true, authentic relationships with people when we are masking our pain and personalities. In turn, people feel more comfortable being vulnerable with us. By being authentic, we teach others that they can also be authentic with us. We give them a safe space to be themselves when we show them that we are being ourselves.

I stay sober by being myself. At first, that self was really messy, erratic, emotionally impulsive, and reckless. Over time, I nurtured that reckless girl. Over more time, I even began liking myself. I like that reckless girl now—she is just less girl and more woman, and a bit more thoughtful and methodical. Just a bit.

That girl needs less external validation now. She needs fewer people surrounding her, but more who are of better quality. The quantity of people in my life dramatically decreased when I stopped drinking, but the quality skyrocketed.

In reality, the people who knew me when I was drinking did not really know me at all, because I never revealed the soft, scared parts of myself. I showed them the girl who didn't care, who was tough, who could drink as much as the boys, and who never got attached to anyone.

But that isn't who I am, even if I wished for so long that it were. I was, and am, the woman who craves connection, and I didn't know how to connect without alcohol. Now, I stay connected by being honest with my feelings and thoughts. That means being honest when I am having good days and bad days. That means not being so worried about how others see me, but making sure I am true to myself.

People can feel the magnetism of authenticity. Let them come or let them go; you need to show the real you now, even if that real you may disappoint them. Most times it, now, people know what they get when they see me. And at all times, I make sure the people I love know that I love them.

Alcohol kept me in a self-destructive but, I thought, self-preserved bubble for a long time. When we ask one person to be in our bubble, the bubble pops, and we realize we do not have to struggle alone. In fact, you cannot get out of the bubble completely by yourself, even if you think you can "outsmart" it. You probably can for a short while, but the time runs out, and alcohol takes its grasp on you, tighter, again.

We are human beings, we need connection. If you have that connection now, lean into it. If you do not have it, start looking for it. People want to help, you deserve the help, and you also deserve to give back to others. Stay connected and you can stay sober.

AMANDA HAAS

Three-times cookbook author. Founder of House of Haas Cooking School. Mom to two teenage boys. Happiest when I don't have to leave the house more than once a day.

Now that I'm almost a year alcohol-free, I'm much more comfortable telling people up front that I'm not drinking. When they ask, "Are you sober?" I simply respond with "I'm not drinking right now."

If I know them well, I go into greater detail about the reason, and it feels good to be honest with them! My favorite thing to say is, "I found alcohol was not serving me, and now that I've taken it out, I don't have any desire to go back."

I don't feel the need to validate other people's ideas about it, including the "Well that's amazing but I'm sure one day you'll feel comfortable having a margarita or a glass of wine again."

When I don't know people well, and I'm going somewhere with them, I'll tell them I'm not drinking and then say something like, "Now you'll always have a driver when we go out!" And then if they don't respond well to that, I don't make plans with them.

Going out feels a lot easier now that I'm more stable in my

sobriety. Because I cook for a living, people assume I'll also drink a lot of wine and cocktails. Instead, I go straight for the bar and put something in my hand, like a soda and lime, or I ask for something yummy that is alcohol-free.

The more I go out, the more I realize most people envy those of us who have given up alcohol. I've found these people are full of questions about how my life has changed and improved. I also stick by the old adage: "If they're judging me, they're not my kind of person!"

I've been very forthcoming about my alcohol recovery. My kids are in their late teens, and I know that my drinking affected them. I try to converse with them about my accomplishments of not drinking. They don't want to talk about it, but they congratulate me. And instead of constantly warning them about the negative effects of alcohol, I'm simply very transparent about how it affected me at their age.

I started binge drinking in high school, and although I was very successful in all the ways you're supposed to be, I often put myself in danger. I try to reiterate that the most important thing is their safety, and that they can always depend on me to come get them if they are in a bad situation with alcohol. And now, they believe me!

I run my business from my home, and I'm the boss, so for a long time I didn't keep any alcohol in my house. But now that I'm more confident and we're always cooking, I'm happy to offer a guest something to drink. Or if I'm gifted wine or champagne, I always regift it to my team to take home and enjoy, as they know I won't need it! I do not judge other people's habits, but I've noticed most people simply won't drink when they're in my home, and I'm fine with that! We just don't make a big deal of it.

I do a ton of work on Instagram Live, and over the past year, people have started asking me why I don't drink. I say the same thing every time, "It wasn't serving me, and now I feel so good I'm not going back!" And because I usually share recipes with them, I offer alcohol-free versions and they are so grateful! Truly, I'm shocked by how many people say, "That's awesome, and I don't drink either!" or "Yeah, I feel so much better when I'm not drinking!" The more we talk about it, the more the stigma is erased.

ANTHONY EDER

Anthony lives in the Midwest. He is living life with intention, hope, and curiosity. He is passionate about self-care, advocating for our voice & purpose, and creating a dance party anywhere he goes. He believes sobriety is a path of self-love and self-discovery. Anthony is a Certified Peer Support Specialist for folks in recovery and struggling with their mental health.

On this Day One, you will wake up and feel like a mess. Your heart will beat fast. You may be consumed with anxiety, shame, and fear. Life feels heavy. It feels so heavy that you don't want to get out of bed.

I understand that you don't want to face the reality of this moment, a moment when you need to ask for help and admit you're struggling. You need to hear me right now ...

You are loved. You are not a bad human. You will rise again from this. I know that feels impossible right now, but your success is possible. I believe in you! This journey will strengthen you, defeat you, challenge you, bless you, and most importantly, teach you. Right now, you are feeling a lot. The emotions are overwhelming, and that's OK.

I know you don't want to be sober and are worried that you

won't belong. It gets better, trust me! You will find your people. You will belong in a loving, safe, and beautiful community. Stay with them.

Go to all the meetings—seriously, go to every meeting that is available. You need connection. You will benefit from hearing other stories of recovery and hope. You will find the most magical humans, the sober queers! They are your foundation and strength. Allow them to hold space for you. Today, you have so many sober friends. It's beautiful, and it's where you feel home.

I also want to remind you to be kind and gentle with yourself. You are carrying a lot, and it feels discouraging, but the hope is that you are doing much better. The work of sobriety continues but your self-awareness and soul are in a better place.

You have the permission to feel. You have the permission to focus on your needs and your priorities. It's not selfish but is an act of self-love and worth. Remember to protect yourself, no matter what. You will want to protect your boundaries, your energy, your time, your heart, and your sobriety. You may feel weird and uncomfortable to speak up and advocate for yourself, but it's worth it. You will feel empowered and free when you do this. It's a life-changing moment for you. You will be proud of yourself today.

Here's another truth for you: You are human and are worthy of new beginnings. You will want to run away and just quit.

Don't quit. Stay. Show up for yourself. Share your heart and vulnerability. Continue to be present for the feelings, the thoughts, and the fears. They will teach you, guide you, and lead you to a stronger you.

You don't have to hold it together all the time. You will learn the value and power of letting go. Right now, let's take a moment to breathe. You ready? Take a breath in, and then breathe out. Keep doing that. Keep breathing. In your breathing, you will find your peace.

You like control. Life is better when it goes your way. You want to everything to be perfect and go smoothly. Well ... today you're still not in control. I know you're rolling your eyes, but you are creating a better relationship with control. You won't control how your sobriety journey will go. You won't have control on how people respond to your sobriety or how they will respond when you create a boundary.

You will also find yourself comparing your sobriety to others. You want what they have. You see their "success" as better or smarter or easier. You will feel frustration when you can't understand the pain, suffering, or doubt. So many things are simply out of your control.

Instead of looking at others, keep the focus on you. Prioritize what you need. What works for others, may not work for you. That's OK. You are figuring it out. Get curious. Try different things. You do have control on how you respond to life. Your power is there. You are badass and it's awesome.

So, let go of control. Take it one day at a time. One breath at a time. There's no need to rush. You will find purpose in the flow. You are making your own waves.

You are knitting, or doing whatever brings you joy, more than you have before, and that has been comforting for you. Keep doing that because it brings you peace and comfort. The activity you love allows you to reflect and connect with your heart, and it provides company for you.

You will also realize that you don't always have to be around people. Surprisingly, you love alone time. It gives you new energy, time to feel, and space to be. You will learn that community with yourself is just as important as having community with others. You will learn the joy in spending time alone. You will learn the freedom in making choices for yourself. Again, just focus on you. You are the center. Make sure to treat yourself well because that's the best gift.

Finally, be open to feedback. Be open to the change. Lean into the discomfort. Welcome this transformation with grace, compassion, and gratitude. Don't lose your joy. Sober joy is real, and you are experiencing it in real time. Commit daily to your sobriety, your needs, and your heart. It matters—*you* matter. You will shine and change lives. Share your story. Share your joy, but share your struggles. Don't hide or be in the closet with sobriety. We've been there before, and we don't need to go back. I see you. I hear you.

I love you. I thank you. I appreciate you deeply. You taught me a lot on this journey. The choice you made today—to get sober—is the best decision you've ever made. Yes, it was hard to make, but in the end this decision will be worth it.

Congratulations! I am proud of you. I am proud of us. May you always know, you are enough, and you belong.

BRENT SELDERS

World traveler with a nomadic spirit. Runner. Entrepreneur. Lover of all sports and dogs. I got sober with the help of Alcoholics Anonymous (AA) on June 10, 2017, and have stayed sober with the help of The Luckiest Club (TLC) since May of 2020.

Q: What has surprised me most about living an alcohol-free life?

A: Freedom

"I always wonder why birds choose to stay in the same place when they can fly anywhere on the earth, then I ask myself the same question," Harun Yahya said.

I was never free when I was drinking. In my mind, I always had an excuse or reason to drink:

Because it is Friday.

I'm going to a baseball game.

Because I'm at a concert.

Thanksgiving? Christmas? Most likely these include family members. I'm *definitely* drinking large amounts of beer, wine, *and* liquor to get through those holidays.

To deal with stress from work.

To pat myself on the back for a job well done.

Because it's Tuesday.

My team won; let's celebrate.

My team lost; I'm mourning.

It helped me get by.

Because it is a beautiful 65-degree spring day.

The day is shitty and snowy. *Drink.*

Thursday night football.

Saturday college football.

NFL Sunday

Monday night Football.

Because I'm stressed.

To get past the things I didn't want to deal with.

I could find a reason for any day and any time I wanted to drink.

I thought I was free at the time. But like a bird with clipped wings, I wasn't getting very far. I was trapped in a cage, in a nasty spiral of drinking and hangovers and starting to ruin relationships. I prioritized alcohol over everything. As a result, I was being a shitty person in the way I treated myself and loved ones. Alcohol controlled my life. Alcohol controlled me.

But I denied that fact.

I can control it, I thought.

I tried to prove this to myself time and time again. Once, after an arrest from a "drunk in public" charge when I was in my late twenties, my lawyer encouraged me to get sober, and then the judge sentenced me to go to 12 AA meetings over two months, which sounded like a death sentence.

So, I quit. No problem. I took six months off from drinking and trained for (and ran) a half marathon. *Two birds with one stone,* I thought. *I don't have an alcohol problem. I can quit anytime I want.*

True alcoholics can't just quit whenever they want.

I put myself in "timeout" from alcohol several other times for various reasons. Once was after less-than-stellar behavior at a friend's wedding. An open bar was a recipe for disaster. And I paid the price for it.

I needed to prove to myself that I could quit drinking without checking myself into rehab to do it. But each time I did these month-long "sobriety stints," I knew I would go back to the bottle. I knew I would go back to binge drinking and blacking out at some point.

For a while, that was my happy place. Until it wasn't anymore.

I realized it was not a happy place at all. It was a deep, dark hole that I could not climb out of—a hole that a three- to six-month sobriety stint would not fix anymore. The alcohol stopped bringing a high, and drinking was not fun anymore. I was stuck.

In June of 2017, I knew it was time to stop drinking for life.

I did not realize the sense of freedom sobriety would give me. I didn't realize the experiences, travels, and people I would get to meet, and connect with. I learned that I could have fun while being sober and remembering *everything.*

The freedom I received from not needing and drinking alcohol has been the greatest gift. I don't need alcohol to get through a Thanksgiving or Christmas with in-laws. I don't need to worry about what I'll do after the seventh inning at a baseball game, and they stop selling beer at the concession stand. Or where I'll go to drink more *after* the concert.

In 2019, I traveled solo to Vietnam and Cambodia. I became hooked on traveling. I loved experiencing new cultures, trying new foods, dancing, smelling the scents, walking the streets, and the overall mystery of where I would end up and what I would see or experience next. I could not have done that had I still been drinking. I would not have trusted myself to make it out of another country alive. A year later I was able to go to South and Central America for the first time.

Now I go to concerts, ball games, weddings, family functions, and other events without having to drink to get through them. I wake up after my team wins a big game without a hangover. And I do the same after a loss, instead of mourning in the bottom of a bottle.

I don't want to paint a perfect picture that life is all sunshine and rainbows and pink clouds as soon as you decide to get sober.

In the beginning, it was extremely tough for me to adjust to such a drastic lifestyle change.

Have I wanted alcohol at times? In the beginning of my sobriety journey, absolutely. My dog passed away when I was six months into sobriety. I wanted to drink so badly. I wanted to pour out a little liquor in memory of him. Then I remembered he thought I was an asshole when I drank. He judged, and rightfully so. I went to a meeting and talked about it. I cried with my girlfriend and my brothers and loved ones. I did not drink that day.

I achieved this newfound freedom through countless AA meetings, step work with my sponsor, TLC meetings, tough conversations, and friendships I made through sobriety communities. It does not happen overnight. And it is 100 percent worth it.

BRUCE EMERD JAMES

Worshipper of my one and only Queen Goddess Lulu. Parent. Seeker of truth, authenticity, awe, and wonder, among so many other things. Creator. Feeler of big feelings. Nature is my religion; my church is the outdoors. Welder, artist, music lover, aspiring author, believer in magic. I want to help men (or anyone, really) be better humans. I am Bruce.

Advice for my Day One self.

If I could sum my advice in a word, that word would be *feelings*. My addiction started as a pleasurable feeling. Then, as the addiction took hold, my goals became about chasing a feeling.

As that feeling became more and more elusive, and the addiction took over, life became about suppressing feelings and forgetting whatever was working over my mind at that moment, along with whatever I was overthinking or whoever had upset my delicate emotional balance.

I would tell myself that we are more than worthy and already more than enough—and, especially, that we are not too much! I would tell myself and others that the feelings and emotions will be big and powerful, because the chemicals we were using narrowed and suppressed and made us forget our feelings. I would tell myself to get ready to experience new and unimaginable emotions as we accrued chemical-free time.

The first time I realized this was about 18 months into my recovery journey. I did not see it at the time, but two seemingly minor events catalyzed the opening of my heart to feel new things, as it had been intended to feel from the beginning.

On an overcast winter day, my four daughters and I were driving an icy, snow-covered mountain road to our local ski resort. As we twisted our way deeper into the canyon, we drove through brief patches of snowfall. In one spot, a strange phenomenon stopped us in our tracks. The giant and delicate flakes of snow slowed in their descent. For a few moments they appeared to almost stop and be suspended in midair.

I pulled my black truck off the main roadway and into a turnout. I looked around for a reason why the snow fell in such an abnormal way. Some distance down the mountain from us, I saw a large, sunny patch where a ray of sunlight was breaking through the cloud ceiling. The gears in my brain began to synchronize, analyzing the reasons of what we saw.

Proud of myself, I opened my mouth to spout off my clever solving of the mystery. As I was about to settle into my oratory groove, my oldest daughter abruptly, gently cut me off saying, "Dad! Shut up and let it be pretty."

I laugh at this memory now, but initially, I was taken aback at the curt statement. However, my silence gave me enough time to get past the surprise and to realize she was right. I did need to just "let it be pretty."

As we sat there quietly, I reached up and turned the key to cut off the engine. For a few minutes, the only sounds were the occasional rustlings of clothing as my daughters shifted for better positions to simply enjoy the beautiful, mystical, magical moment.

It would certainly not be possible to take my Day One self and somehow describe the awe and wonder of that moment in a way that does it justice. Even now, it is impossible to fully convey all of those real-time emotions and what they caused my body and mind and soul to feel in that liminal space there with my four lovely daughters.

As I wrote this, I received a text message from my stepmom. She let me know that my grandfather had passed. This was not a surprise. Ever since Grandma passed six years ago, he has been on the decline. She was his reason to live. He was so devoted to her that in the last several years of her life, he would graciously turn down our invitations to go hunting or fishing on the slight chance that Grandma might need him during the day.

After Grandma passed, we were able to get him out a couple of more times. He even harvested a moose at the age of 89 on his last hunting excursion. The only picture I have is one of him crouched in a hunker with a smile of pure joy on his face. And as a testament to his taking care of himself, he could still stand unassisted from that position!

I knew the man for just over half of his life and in all that time, I never witnessed him shout or express his anger in an unhealthy way. The worst thing I ever heard him say, with a relaxed and even tone, was, "Well ... the man ain't worth killin' or someone already would've done it." And his typical insulting idioms, "Well, he's a prince of a fellow." Or "I gotta say, he's a different breed of cat."

This relates to my Day One self because I would tell me that my mind would slowly clear up. Memories will bubble up at times when we need to revisit them. We will be able to recognize complex emotions in someone else and understand their perspective at a deeper level since chemicals and their sticky residues no longer cloud our brain and affect the physiology of the endocrine system as hormones regain equilibrium.

In those days, I would never have experienced the loving memories I have of my grandfather. In fact, I would most likely have been using more heavily to quell the grief and pain. But with a clear mind, a clean and properly functioning body, I can sit with the grief, sorrow, pain, loss, frustration, sadness—and the joy, happiness, relief, and peace ... *all* the of complex feelings that come with the loss of a dear, dear loved one. I would tell my Day

One self, "We get to feel all of that now, and we don't have to be ashamed of feeling all those emotions."

As my Day One self sat next to me, listening, and becoming overwhelmed, I would tell me that along with the growing complexity we feel during these other two instances, we will get to experience the most exquisite emotional complexity of all: love. Without the chemicals fucking up our brain and body, we would get to feel our heart burst open and sing at the sight of someone who is more than our soulmate. This emotion is often romanticized, the "one in a million" or a "once in a lifetime love," but we found something even greater because our eyes were clear and free. We found our one—our *one completely.*

I had joined a private sobriety group on Facebook at the invitation of the group's founder, a prominent stand-up comedian and content creator who had also had an irregularly scheduled livestream centered around conversations on sobriety and support. A few weeks into my being in the group, a new name appeared, commenting on a post. Clicking on her name to open her profile, and seeing her picture, I froze. My world stopped spinning for just a moment.

A thick beanie obscured her head, and aviator sunglasses covered much of her face. Even though I could only see a smile and dark golden hair loosely falling across the collar of her puffy black coat, my heart leapt in my chest and sent a wave of energy that I felt from my hair to my toenails. After I caught my breath and recovered, a vibration was left humming in my soul.

Seeing her picture awakened my heart. And it would send out that wave of energy each time something new occurred—her first "like" of a comment I made; her first response to a comment I made; her responding with a GIF of Hermione Grainger hugging Harry Potter—in my mind, I saw her hugging me and I felt it in my body; the first time she reached out to me through Messenger; offering me her phone number after we had messaged for a few weeks; sending me a song that made her think of me; our first phone conversation; our first video chat and seeing her sparkling eyes and gorgeous whole face for the first time; the first "I love you."

We live 1,248 miles apart. For the first five months, our relationship was formed across digital signals of Wi-Fi and cellular service. We waited almost six months before we met in person. And those were brief meetings. We shared a few hours across a few days before she would return to her house, and I would return to the room-share I had rented. But we took walks, we ate a breakfast sitting on the bank of the beautiful river. But that first meeting, the first time I could look at her with nothing between us but free air and be close enough to touch ... in that moment, I was so overwhelmed with love and all its divine and indescribably beautiful complexities, that I literally could not stand.

I felt my knees begin to buckle and had to sit before I fell down the steps of the walking path bridge where we had agreed to meet. My glorious, joyful tears washed her hands as I let the emotions flow out from within me.

"I wanted so badly to play this cool, but I knew in my soul that I would fail miserably at it," I said with a breaking voice. Thirty months later (and still long distance for now), she still makes me weak in the knees when I look into her eyes.

We understand that we are taking a non-traditional and slow route in this society of immediate gratification and the rush into physical relationships. But we also know that we are doing this thing the right way by building on a foundation of emotional connection and learning communication and attachment styles.

We each have a constant desire to grow and improve ourselves so we each bring our best self to the team and partnership. She still twists my belly with butterflies when I think of her, and we are excited beyond description as we anticipate what the future is bringing.

I would wrap it up with helping my Day One self understand that these few instances are just the beginning. The best is yet to come. I would tell me that we were sleepwalking through life, and even though our heartfelt dead and withered, we could think of it as a wintering season—that spring was just right around the corner and just hidden from view. And that with that inevitable awakening, our consciousness would increase, our heart would be jolted back to life, and it would sing. We would see beauty and miracles in the most unexpected places.

I'd tell myself that our life would change is such a way that the variety and depth of feelings would be unimaginable and indescribable. I would tell me that we would feel safe enough with a goddess teammate that we would surrender our heart to her completely and experience a love that grows and expands each day —that we will wake loving her more each morning and fall more deeply in love with her with each breath that fills our lungs. That we would find our purpose and take steps to move in its direction. Despite how hopeless and dead we felt, there was, in fact, hope. We would learn how to truly find heart space and *live!*

CHRISTA C. LOMBARDI

Shy girl turned public relations executive working and playing hard in New York City. Traded "No Pain, No Champagne" workout tank for an "Alcohol-Free AF" tank in January 2020. Found freedom joining The Luckiest Club (TLC) and openly sharing my experiences with anxiety, depression, disordered eating, and sobriety. Now living in Boston, where I'm a book hoarder and dog mom to Rigby.

This One's for the Shy Girls
    By Christa Lombardi

"Christa?"

Mrs. Rowan stands before our first-grade classroom, her voice climbing a full octave as she calls out my name. She offers me a gentle smile that reaches her eyes—warm, brown eyes now wide with surprise. She is not the only one taken aback. Even I am surprised to find my own hand up.

"Yes," I reply softly.

My hand is not raised like the other children with their arrow-straight arms outstretched and fingertips wiggling.

No, my right arm is raised in a soft bend—a hesitant, protective position that I know all too well. I've spent my young life embroiled in a private game of tug-of-war: my longing to shine and connect at constant odds with my deep-seated fear of being fully seen and heard. It is hard to be the shy girl with the softly bent arm, the one who is routinely stuck between shooting her arm straight up and keeping it glued to her side.

I had just volunteered to participate in my school's talent show, an event where I'd shock everyone by taking the stage in a shiny red unitard and cowgirl hat to side-step along to Escape Club's "Wild, Wild West."

Yes, me—the nice, shy girl who was constantly told by her classmates, "Christa, you're sooooo quiet."

Every year at back-to-school conferences, teachers would confirm how bright I was, yet reiterate that I really should speak up more. My mom remained my fierce advocate, reassuring teachers that my introspective style was a positive trait. But each morning on the school bus, I'd grip the ripped, plastic seats as my stomach fluttered with nerves and my body zapped with anxiety. I worried that I was different than other kids and wondered if something was wrong with me. They didn't seem to have the same persistent thoughts warning them to stay quiet. I wondered: *Why does it constantly feel so scary to vocalize my thoughts and feelings?*

Being the "shy girl" came with an endless rush of deep, overpowering emotions—happiness, sadness, anger, fear, anxiety, and excitement—which crashed and swirled together, culminating in an uncomfortable energy peak that permeated my mind and body. This energy monster suffocated me. It kept me quiet and disconnected. It taught me how to be lonely, because it told me I was the only person who could feel the way I did. By the age of five, I was already learning how to fight the monster.

Dance was my first intoxicant—a way to find fleeting relief from the energy monster. I felt the internal shift whenever I stepped foot inside the ballet studio and began to move my body through the familiar positions and routines. The movement quieted my brain and worrying thoughts, and every chaîné, arabesque, or plié felt like a new language of sorts. Through dance, I'd found a safe way to communicate the confusing thoughts and emotions swirling inside of me. The girl with the softly bent arm in a classroom found a way to be seen and heard in the dance studio.

Outside the dance studio, I found escape through books and worthiness through praise. I strove to be "good" in all areas of my life: to be the best listener and kindest friend, to achieve high test scores, and to follow all the rules at home. I believed that if I did everything just right, I could make my anxiety go away.

The harder I tried to fix my inner world through external validation, the more disconnected I became. With puberty came the belief that not only was my mind not right, but now my body was not right either. By fourth grade, I'd already envisioned a new, improved version of myself: "I want a thin, tan body and curly hair," I typed into my electronic diary.

By the time I was in high school, when my inner world felt so wild, I grew addicted to the control I had over my food and figure. I relished the recognition I received for my physical changes—until the praise turned to worried whispers as my body kept shrinking.

I felt a growing distance between me and my peers, which increased as they began to experiment with alcohol. I feared that if I drank, it would hurt my family and cause me to lose my "good girl" status, which provided a sense of validation. I graduated from high school with honors and received scholarships based on essays I wrote about my choice to not drink alcohol.

I don't remember the exact moment I changed my mind about alcohol; I'd made it through my whole first semester away at college without experimenting with this substance.

But my first sip was unforgettable: the tingle of pale, citrusy bubbles down my throat and the warm glow that quickly overcame me. As we huddled inside the dorm room, swigging from our malt beverage bottles, it was as though I'd suddenly discovered what I'd been missing. Alcohol assured me that I did belong and know how to connect. It promised me an easier way to be in the world, and it granted me a temporary reprieve from my shyness, anxiety, and body image struggles.

I'd found my new intoxicant, and it was more potent than dancing had ever been. It only took one night for me to learn that I never wanted to live without alcohol again.

For the rest of college, alcohol and I joined forces—and were a force to be reckoned with. My social life took off, but I managed to maintain impressive grades, write for the school paper, volunteer in a nursing home, and play club field hockey. I landed three great internships, and after graduation, scored my dream job at a large public relations agency. I showed up in New York City with both an ambitious nature and a party-girl persona—two things that would set the stage for what was to come.

In 2015, after I'd spent nearly a decade of working and playing hard, life in the city began to take a toll on my well-being. I received diagnoses of major depressive disorder and generalized anxiety disorder, and I took a medical leave from work.

When I returned, I felt a renewed sense of energy and was hopeful for a fresh start. I was now on medication and further supported myself with weekly therapy appointments. I was relieved that I was back to "normal."

I was surprised and dismayed when my depression and anxiety crept back by 2016, but I was too embarrassed to tell anyone. For the first time, I began to wonder if I was drinking too much. I began taking the "Am I an Alcoholic?" quizzes and reading women's addiction and recovery memoirs.

Over the next four years, I practiced moderating my drinking. I'd worked so hard to create this new "improved" version of me— the confident, popular one who was no longer known as a shy girl —and I realized how much pain was buried underneath. I'd become a person who never let anyone see who she really was inside. I was terrified of letting go of alcohol—the one thing that I believed transformed me into the person everyone else wanted me to be.

Nobody told me I had to let it go. I didn't have a DUI. I didn't lose my job or my family or my home. From the outside, I may have even seemed to be living my best life. My mind twisted itself inside out debating whether I needed to quit drinking.

Finally, after years of uncertainty, I read a chapter in Laura McKowen's book about drinkers asking ourselves the "wrong damn question." As Laura writes, the real question we should ask ourselves is, "Am I free?"

For me, the answer was a loud "NO."

At that moment, I was ready to finally listen to what I knew I needed, even if others questioned my decision. In January 2020, I chose to let go of alcohol and to use my voice and my words to share my journey. I posted screenshots from an app that tracked my alcohol-free days on my social media channels, and wrote about emotions I was experiencing, alcohol-free beverages I was trying, and tips for navigating social events without alcohol. In April 2020, I was featured in an *InStyle* article about staying sober during a global pandemic. My choice to break the stigma about mental health struggles and sobriety in these public ways later led to speaking engagements at my workplace.

As I write this, I am approaching three years of sobriety. I am in the same Jersey City apartment, but everything else in my life is different. Before I quit drinking, staring out my floor-to-ceiling windows at the New York City skyline made me feel lonely and separate from everyone else. It reminded me how every day I would put on my best happy face and go into the city to work and go out with friends, but I would come home, cry, and write in my journals about my struggles with alcohol and wanting to die. Now when I look at the skyline, I smile because it's become a recognizable backdrop for my "shares" in The Luckiest Club, my online sobriety support group. It reminds me how, meeting-by-meeting, I practiced letting other people truly see me and all of my dimensions—not just my happy face. These people have witnessed my sadness, my anger, my joy, my anxiety, and my excitement, and they continue to hold space for me exactly as I am.

I'm not sure what the future holds for me, and that makes me a little uncomfortable. But I do know I have never felt so connected and loved as I do right now. Today I am freer to be me than I've ever been, and this knowledge causes my spirit to dance.

ALEKS L.

Sober Warrior. Cat Mom. Enneagram 4. Therapist. Midwesterner, specifically, Chicagoland.

The interesting thing about getting sober is that I knew early on that I had an unhealthy relationship with alcohol. Having severe complex anxiety, my brain constantly reacted to noise, fear, threats, and intrusive thoughts. Alcohol was the one thing that let me have some sort of respite from what seemed like an endless cycle of distress.

Part of my resistance to getting sober was acknowledging that removing alcohol from my life meant I didn't have the escape valve that alcohol provided. Getting sober meant that I would have to experience my anxiety in its purest form—and that seemed unbearable.

I held onto alcohol as my way to maintain my peace of mind from my anxiety. Taking back control over the anxiety that I did not choose to have, felt like a loss of control all on its own.

My struggle with my mental health, to a great degree, drove me to not want to or be able to put down alcohol for good. I didn't want to live in depression, anxiety, trauma, and low self-esteem, so I lived in the bottle instead. Alcohol has a strange and terrifying way to create a place that feels safe and warm. It is temporary relief in exchange for long-term suffering. It would take me a long time to learn that the short-term discomfort of sitting with my emotions would give me the long-term freedom that my authentic self-craved.

My therapist caught on quickly to my unhealthy patterns. She initially said, "Give me 30 days of continuous sobriety, and I'll drop it."

So, I did. And then picked right back up on day 31. This was my way to prove that I didn't have a problem, to continue to live in a state of quasi-denial regarding the grip alcohol now had on my life. Alcohol was what I thought about early in the morning, during my breaks at work, and the thing I waited patiently—and somewhat impatiently—to rip into after a long day at work.

I started my weekend mornings with alcohol and stretched my drinking into the afternoon and evening to give myself two days of relief from the stress and anxiety I held onto during the week. I hid alcohol in my bedroom, in the living room, wherever I needed to have easy access during family dinners. I learned how to manage my behavior while intoxicated so nobody could tell. I became good at hiding my addiction.

I thought drinking helped me be a better friend and to show my appreciation to others. My "tell" that I was drunk eventually became the long, loving, emotional, sappy text messages that I sent to my friends and cousin telling them how wonderful they were and how grateful I was for them.

At first, the responses were comfy cozy. Eventually the response became, "You have a ride home, right?"

I thought alcohol made me funny, as my friends and I would laugh the next morning reading through our drunken exchanges. I feared that giving up alcohol would strip me of these qualities, that I would become less fun, less funny, less entertaining. I worried that people would no longer want to spend time with me, and I couldn't stand the thought of not having my people near me and available to me.

I was 20-something, and alcohol was the centerpiece at every event. The social pressure to drink regularly kept me away from sobriety for a long time. I crave social connection, and all my friends, professional events, and life events involved alcohol in one way or another. I didn't want to be left out or feel disconnected—or, even more importantly, shamed.

We seem to live in a world where *not drinking* labels us as the "odd one out." Something is "wrong with us" or we are "no longer fun" if we don't drink. The fear of being shunned and judged for my history of drinking—or my current lack thereof—kept me in fear and avoiding the sobriety I desperately needed. When I got sober, I did lose certain connections that were held together by alcohol. I still sometimes question if I miss the people or if my drinking self misses the opportunity to check out.

In my drinking, I functioned at exceptional levels. This made it a lot more challenging to admit that I needed to give up alcohol when I couldn't see the negative effects all around me. I heard of people who would get fired or in accidents or lose relationships. None of those things happened to me (somehow). I finished graduate school with a 4.0 GPA. I excelled professionally, landing a fellowship at a highly respected organization. I learned and grew and appeared to thrive in others' eyes.

If I could do all of these things, then I certainly had no problem with alcohol. If I had a problem, I assumed, my life would have fallen apart.

I wish I could say that none of my sobriety-related fears ever came true. But in reality, I did lose friends. I did face judgment. I had to work harder to connect socially and find the places where I belong. Sobriety had costs. It also had benefits that far surpassed my wildest imagination.

While getting sober, I found a community of other sober humans. These connections I formed were deep, fun, compassionate, and genuine. I found the connections I was trying to foster while I was drinking but was incapable of creating. I didn't know that the sober friendships I was making were the exact type of relationships I desperately craved.

I got to witness others' growth in sobriety and cheer them on or help hold them up when they struggled. I gained friends outside of my sober community, too. I could show up for people in the ways they needed. I was able to ask for help in the way I needed. Moreso, I actually knew what I needed. I began walking away with less and less resentment from interactions that didn't provide what I needed.

I shed shame. I thought something was incredibly wrong with me that led me to drink. I didn't want my medical providers to see me as an addict. I didn't want people to whisper about my short-comings behind my back. I feared that getting sober would immediately highlight every last thing that was wrong with me, and I would never be able to recover from the slander that would come with my acknowledging my struggle.

In sobriety, however, I found power in putting alcohol down. My sober self embraced imperfection, owned my story, and saw my rebellion against alcohol as a source of strength, pride, dignity, and achievement.

I no longer feel shame for having struggled. My journey with alcohol is just another part of my story. It doesn't make me any better or worse than any other person who has or has not been in a nasty relationship with booze.

Most importantly, I gained freedom. When I drank to squash my anxiety and depression, this gave me a false sense of freedom. Getting sober and doing the exceptionally hard work required to maintain sobriety gave me true freedom from having a disorder, an emotion, a situation, an interaction, or a substance run my life.

I didn't know this freedom existed until I was willing to face fear, go screaming into the abyss, and come out the other side with a life I actually want to be present for.

Wherever you are on your journey, I hope you know, you are worthy of the gifts and freedom of sobriety.

JAMISON MILLER

Father, single dad of two. Chicken herder and cat wrangler who's 46. Runner, social justice advocate, wood tinkerer. Childhood sexual abuse survivor. The last one to leave the party, regular blackout-er.

My first memory of not feeling right about drinking happened in my mid-twenties when I noticed that despite telling myself not to, I couldn't drive home from work without stopping for a six-pack of beer.

Having a hangover on a given morning, I'd say, "Good grief, I'm going to take the night off tonight."

After lunch though, I'd feel better, and the first sparks of drinking again would begin trickling in. In the final hours of work, I would get more forceful with my self talk, "No way, not tonight. I just need to get some sleep."

I was rarely successful. Almost every evening, the craving would take hold, and I could easily let go of the memory of how I'd felt that morning.

I murmured an "It's not that bad," or "I'll drink lots of water with it tonight," or "I don't have to drink all of them," or any other phrases I could use to console my guilt and shame of not being able to follow through with a night off.

If I were ever invited to a happy hour, to hang out at a bar, to go to a live show—any social event that included alcohol at all—I would definitely throw out any intention of not drinking. When I was drinking with others, my shame evaporated because I wasn't hiding it, the way I did when I drank alone. I barely let myself notice that my craving to drink was more regular than my social engagements, and I barely let myself notice that I was drinking alone more than with others.

I definitely didn't allow myself to notice just how much I was drinking. By the time I entered my thirties, I was well on the path of hiding the extent of my drinking from everyone—especially myself.

My denial of my issues with drinking was rooted in self-deception that took on several forms.

Hiding the behavior. As I progressed in my addiction, I began to drink on my own before and/or after I was out with others. On one hand, this caused little trouble or stress when I was single, as I had the privacy to do so without others knowing. But I was still embarrassed because, of course, I knew about it and knew I was drinking more than I wanted to.

When I was married, hiding extra drinking was much more stressful. I had to mask extra alcohol purchases, hide stashes, and dispose of empties. And of course, I needed to disguise my altered state. I introduced so much lying, and thus suspicion, into the relationship.

How did I do that over the course of years? I lied to myself about it. Each time I managed to get through another cycle of inebriation, I pretended it hadn't happened. The times I did confront the reality of my experience, I told myself it wouldn't happen again.

Hiding from feelings. After some time in sobriety and working with a therapist, I have come to understand and recognize how I was feeling when a craving would come on and why I felt such soothing relief from alcohol. Drinking alcohol almost immediately calmed anxiety, fear, self-consciousness, and so on. This amounted to my kind of hiding from these feelings, and when I hid from them, I only postponed dealing with them—they didn't go away. This hiding and fear response to strong, or even just uncomfortable, feelings no doubt stems from some of my childhood experiences and was a coping mechanism I couldn't sustain any longer.

Dissociation. Sometimes, even after months of sobriety, I would experience dissociation or losing touch with an awareness of myself or my surroundings. This was another coping mechanism that likely arose from childhood trauma but came up in ways that facilitated drinking or a relapse. Much like lying to myself to hide my drinking from others, when I dissociated, I felt like I was hiding what was happening right in front of me from myself. I've heard others refer to this as a zombie-like experience. I found myself putting beer or wine in my shopping cart, or stopping at a liquor store, without fully engaging with the behavior. It was another way for my brain to continue getting the drug without my pesky conscience getting in the way.

I also supported my denial by noting that no one besides my partner had a problem with my drinking. This is tricky, as I have learned that our codependent relationship was always cycling around my drinking and her trying to control it. It was an unhealthy relationship. However, for years I felt a good deal of anger towards her because she was the only one complaining about my drinking.

In time, I saw that this was, in large part, because she was the only real witness to the extent of my behavior. I could hide it from others. When I did start to honestly tell other people about my patterns and experiences, I learned that it wasn't my partner's problem, but mine.

So perhaps not surprisingly, a key turning point in my sobriety journey was a shift towards being open, straight, and honest with myself. Crucially, that honesty could not be in a self-harming voice, could not be about beating myself up, could not be judgmental. Through practice and in time, I learned to approach honesty with myself as a nurturing and comforting form of self-care. I had to learn to be with myself in a kind and loving way. This helped me begin to see my patterns without shame and establish a life from which I didn't want to use alcohol to escape.

JASON GREEN

I am a husband to Amanda, Dad to my "very good boy" Blue, and love playing and watching sports. I particularly enjoy playing golf and discovered that my game got much better when I quit drinking. I never thought I could be social without alcohol.

Dear Jason,

I'm not sure if you will even read this, because you are probably too busy reaching for the next drink or sleeping off a terrible hangover from the night before. That's OK. I know you are going through a rough time and are struggling to find a way out of this mess you have gotten yourself into.

Again, it's OK. I want you to know that this is the hardest thing you will ever go through, but you will heal, in time. I know you have tried dozens of ways to heal, but you just didn't figure it out at first that you couldn't do it alone. But you do find healing in a wonderful community of others whose thing is alcohol.

Now, let me tell you what is so great and surprising about living in sobriety, because I know you can't even imagine it at this time.

You will be surprised at how much more enjoyable life is when you aren't constantly numbing yourself with alcohol. I know you drank so much of the time because life was "boring" or "mundane." Trust me, it is infinitely more enjoyable than you can imagine. What is "boring" is experiencing every day of your life in a fog of an alcohol-induced haze, numbing your feelings, and then spending a lot of your time in bed or on the couch trying to get over a hangover.

The mornings will have more meaning when you get a good night's rest, with that first cup of hot coffee that you enjoy along with breakfast that you don't have to worry about keeping down. The sunrises are amazing, the cool crisp air is refreshing, and the endless possibilities of a new day before you are exciting. Even those mornings when life seems to be a struggle, and it's hard to get out of bed and face the day are infinitely better without alcohol getting in the way.

You will be surprised at so many things, moments, and events that you will experience without the cloud of alcohol hanging over you. You will go to your first concert without alcohol, and remember every single part of it. You will go on an amazing 15-day cruise overseas without drinking and experience so many other parts of the world without walking around in a fog. Sporting events, birthday parties, and just having dinner with friends will be so much more interesting and memorable simply because, well, you remember them.

I know right now you face a lot of depression and anxiety. And that's OK. Trust me, it is OK to not be OK. And while a big reason why you drink is to deal with this anxiety and depression, which really just makes it worse. You will need to work to address these issues without alcohol, but you will learn that it gets better.

It was definitely surprising to realize how many other people also struggle with anxiety and alcohol, and they will be a tremendous support in helping you to deal with this. Another big surprise: You will learn how to meditate and journal and actually enjoy it! These really help you with your anxiety.

And the most surprising thing about living a sober life is how many new friendships you will forge by joining a community of others who struggle with alcohol. I know you keep hearing people say, "If they can do it, then you can do it." And you think that it is impossible for you to do this. Well, you are half correct. It is impossible for you to do it—by yourself.

I know you have searched for a group that can help you with your struggles, and you will eventually find that group. And people in the group will care for you and support you without any judgment. You will be surprised at how open and supportive these people are. You will enjoy spending time with them and supporting them as you heal—and then help others heal. We do get better!

Finally, the last thing that surprised me most about living a sober life was how many of your friends and family will support you and love you for making this decision. Contrary to what you may believe, making this change does not mean then end of your life; it means it is really just beginning.

You will discover that your friends really love you for being *you*, and not because of the person you think you are when you drink. You do not have to drink to have fun and for people to enjoy being around you. Sometimes your friends and family don't really like to be around you when you drink. They have to constantly worry about you and make sure that you don't do anything to hurt yourself, or others. Trust me, they don't really care that you aren't drinking. You seem to think that others are drinking as much as you are, but they aren't. And you start to realize this when you live a sober life.

In short, everything about your life becomes better in sobriety. Life is not perfect, it never is. You will have ups and downs, but you are now in a much better position to handle the down days that you would by reaching for a drink. Even at the end of your roughest days, when you can lie your head on the pillow at night, sober and clear headed, that is a win. And you can be of service by sharing your story and helping others. That gives you so much fulfillment and enjoyment.

I will leave you with this: Sobriety is hard work. It takes time, so please be patient with yourself. It is hard, but it is worth it. As we say in recovery, this is not your fault, but it is your responsibility. And you cannot do it alone. Keep going. Keep showing up, and never give up on yourself. You are worth it. And you are loved.

JEFFREY LARSON GRAHAM

Father of four. Mechanical engineer and former offensive lineman for the University of Cincinnati Bearcats. Creator of GettingBAC2zero and the men's group TakeitBAC. Contributor through @bac.2.zero. An expert with sharing bad dad jokes.

Maybe I would've stopped earlier if I had known.

I knew it was over the night I could not scrounge up another lie or another excuse. The fight was over and all I could do was sit there and take the barrage of aggravation she repeated from so many nights before.

I searched frantically for an unused lie or a forgotten excuse, but I found none. It was over, I had lost. I was mentally and physically exhausted and could not find the strength to fight back any longer. My drinking days were done—the 55-year run I had traveled hand-in-hand with alcohol was over, and so was life, as I saw it.

The drinking was a thing of the past, but so was the fun, the confidence, the laughs and the ability to navigate life without going crazy. I was destined to live without alcohol but was also destined to live life without life. Or so I thought.

Alcohol had been my answer. From that day when I was able to walk through that high school party feeling like I belonged to the day when I bought that last 12-pack to manage the day's stress, alcohol was my "go to" for everything from the great moments that we celebrated together to the sheer panic of the anxiety attacks that it helped me through. Alcohol was not just a luxury; it was as crucial to life as oxygen is for survival. And alcohol meant survival for me. To think about facing the day without drinking, was enough to make me want to drink ... so I did!

Three years ago, sobriety was not a choice for me. I had run out of the options that make choosing a luxury. Sobriety was a last resort, and I made the decision only because I was on the verge of losing everything that meant anything to me.

I had burned up my allotted tomorrows and was finally faced with the reality of today. I could either accept something that I prayed to avoid for so long, or lose my family, my career, my health, and my freedom.

I did not *want* to be sober, but life had backed me into a corner with one way out—a life free from the one thing that made my life doable. I didn't want sobriety. I wanted to somehow become the first person to walk this earth who could take only certain parts of the package that alcohol brought with its deceitful promises. My choices were unhappiness or a life without happiness ... or so I thought.

My recovery began in those rooms. I had received my penance and was sentenced to live as "one of them" with only cigarettes and coffee as my sources of pleasure. The days of freedom were behind me, and my life was now subject to weekly meetings with a room full of "I told you so."

I wasn't one of them; I was different. I hadn't wrecked the car; I never wore the silver bracelets, lost a job, or had to walk on a straight line while reciting the alphabet. I was just a guy who worked his butt off during the day, provided for his family, and earned the right to drink at night. I deserved to drink. It was the thing that allowed me to do it all again in the morning.

I didn't live in a tent under a bridge; I was taking care of business and earning the right to "unwind" with 24 to 28 beers per night! Right?

I was angry that sobriety was happening to me, I didn't deserve it. Sobriety was a death sentence. It meant the end of living, not in the sense of a beating heart, but living life with a full spectrum of emotions.

The light was red. It was time to stop. It was time to stop drinking and enjoying life. How can you have fun in life when you take away the one thing that you truly believe makes life fun to begin with? Drinking stopped, but that meant that the life I wanted to feel was ending too ... or so I thought.

In the early months of my sobriety, I learned to live without alcohol. I learned to work, I learned to socialize. I learned to deal with life, and I also learned to accept that life without alcohol was dull. That first year of living alcohol-free was hard, but more than anything, it was uncomfortable. I had to learn that I could deal with life by myself.

Life was returning to a new norm, and I even found that I could enjoy things, but with an asterisk. I realized that socializing was fun, that concerts were fun, and that special occasions were fun, but with an asterisk. Yes, they were enjoyable, but the asterisk referred to the fact that I wasn't drinking.

Life with an asterisk was good, but not as good as it could be without that asterisk attached. Concerts were fun, parties were fun, even tailgating before a big game was fun, but I wasn't drinking, so it was only as fun as is possible without booze ... or so I thought.

I had joined an online support group called The Luckiest Club, where people like me got together and shared about their lives. It was a group where all of "us" who were all similarly sentenced to life without alcohol could get together with our own kind and pretend to smile. The other members had the smiles, and surprisingly, some of them looked convincing.

I attended those meetings as an observer until I began to notice something changing inside. I was getting the tools that I needed to help me "not" drink, but I also began to receive an unanticipated gift that I never expected: I began to believe.

I always felt it's hard to believe in something you don't believe in. And I certainly didn't believe in a life after alcohol. But they did ... The people behind the same faces that I saw daily on Zoom did something for me that I was unable to do for myself—they believed in me when I couldn't. They carried the load and walked me down a path of belief until I could finally begin to do it for myself.

These familiar strangers believed that life could be what I just knew wasn't possible, and they allowed me to taste it and live it with their help until I was able to do it alone. For that I will be eternally grateful. Their smiles were real, their laughter was genuine and their zest for life was surprisingly possible in a life that should have been a red-light world.

They were living in green, and their sentences didn't end with an asterisk, but with a big bold exclamation point. Their belief in themselves and the belief they had in me were enough. Because of them, I tried. Because of them I opened my mind and my heart to allow the possibilities to come in. Because of them, I was able to release the parking brake that I had angrily applied, and they gave me enough belief to let the clutch out.

The light turned green!

I remember the night I first realized that I could live asterisk-free. We had gone to a sports bar to see a local singer play. I was surrounded by others who were drinking and enjoying the evening as I'd always done the past. Suddenly, I realized that I was laughing, enjoying music, and living an evening of pure joy without an asterisk. I was laughing like I'd always done, and I was doing everything I had done before—but without alcohol.

The asterisk was gone, and in its place was *my* belief. It wasn't a chosen belief, it wasn't a fake belief, and it wasn't a forced belief. It was a fact. I was living life like I had believed never to be possible again. I was not craving alcohol, I was not missing alcohol, and I wasn't living with an asterisk. The light was green.

Sobriety is not my death sentence; it is not the end of me. Life without alcohol is a freedom from chains and shackles that I never knew I wore. Life without alcohol has given me back the ability to dream like I once did, to anticipate like a child at Christmas, to feel things that were once just words on paper.

My life is mine. I am no longer living on alcohol's terms, but on mine. I am no longer on alcohol's schedule, splitting my time with family, friends, and my own personal goals with something that gives me nothing but long-term regret.

Life without alcohol has given me back my pride and my self-worth and a desire to do more than just exist. Life is mine, and I can now choose how I want to live it. It all started with belief that it was possible. And it all started with a group of familiar strangers who believed for me until I could believe for myself. If you are one of them, and if you're in this book, I'm sure you are ... thanks!

www.facebook.com/groups/bac2zero

jeff@gettingbac2zero.com

JESSI BRICKNER

Resides in Las Vegas, Nevada, with husband, two huskies and a pug. Now a mortgage loan originator and passionate about volunteering with the Trauma Intervention Program of Southern Nevada. Lover of 90-day fiancé, housewives, and crime shows. An imperfectly balanced Libra. Sobriety date: February 15, 2019

Early in sobriety I didn't know how to support myself. My loved ones were over my bullshit, and a lot of trust needed to be built up again. It was rough.

I didn't know on a day-to-day basis if I was still going to have a relationship or not because of the bridges I burned. I had to be selfish about *me*. In order for me to regain trust, I had to stay on the course. I went to work, walked my dogs, went to meetings, and continuously focused on getting better and doing nothing else. I told my significant other, "I am doing what I need to do to get this to work."

A good bit of my heavy drinking career was jam-packed with bullshit excuses, hiding, and lies about drinking. I lost an awful bit of trust and in order to regain that trust, I needed to be truthful and patient. Tears were shed, and I was pissed off about all the questions my significant other constantly threw at me. Why should he trust me? I swore up and down I would get better only to come home from work buzzed after every shift. I had to get angry and competitive and look forward to the day he would see me prove him wrong.

I set barriers around meetings that would help gain sobriety. That was my priority. I realized he even felt a jealousy about the meetings. He tried and tried to tell me I had a problem, and I told him off and told him he was wrong—only to now prioritize my day around meetings and look forward to taking support from complete strangers. I think any person who loves us and has not been punched with a reliance on a substance will not understand.

It was time to be honest. I had to tell him that people at the meeting were just like me. They told me they, too, thought they could just have one. They told me they had also tried to stop on their own, and it didn't work. And last but not least, they told me if I just kept coming back, it would get better.

I invited him to come to a meeting and see what it was like. That opened a whole new door. Though he never went to a meeting with me, it showed him that I was willing to make him a part of this, and I was not hiding anything from him.

Once the dust settled and trust was working its way back into the household, I began to realize that in order for me to be supported, I needed to support as well. It was time for me to again get honest with what I was going through. Newton's third law states: "For every action, there is an equal but opposite reaction."

I can't help but believe that if I require support, so do my loved ones. They need to learn how to care for me, and I need to learn what they need from Sober Jessi. Do I owe an apology for anything I put a loved one through? I owe them my assurance that I plan on doing so much better, and in order for this plan to work, I have to explain boundaries and what I need.

Action: This is what I need. Reaction: What do you need? Where have I not shown up in a place you needed me before?

I then read Laura McKowen's teachings about "The pregnancy principle"—treat your sobriety like a precious baby that you need to nurture. My loved ones didn't need to hear about it, but I could surely make them comfortable being around my precious new life. Many people I've come across in the rooms have a hard time with this and will accommodate friends' needs over putting their sobriety into danger.

I am not better than anyone, and I don't think there is a right or wrong answer, but I needed to take my time and build my boundaries and toolbox. For instance, I was to go on a European cruise down the Danube River shortly into my sober journey. I had to cancel it because there was no way I would get through this without being riddled with temptation to grab a nice glass of wine while soaking in sights of my favorite countries.

It is also my responsibility to remember life still goes on for people, and I do not need them to change their events or guilty pleasures just to make me happy. I can root them on while they go to gorgeous vineyards and have stunning meals with savory cocktails. I do not have to go along for the ride. If I do go, I let my significant other or an attendee know that when I get anxious or have enough, I have my escape plan. That way they can understand that when I take off, everything is fine. I just have to go protect the precious and vulnerable new life.

It is most important for me to stay in my lane. This is my journey. My loved ones are a part of the tour, but I am the assistant guide, and my higher power is in charge.

We can make things so much more complicated than they need to be. I find life is easiest when I accept the cards I am dealt and share with my loved ones what I am going through. Nobody knows to be supportive if they can't see the storm. However, when I remain my biggest supporter and nurture my "precious new life" things all flow together magically.

I am supported. I am loved.

KATHLEEN HOPPER PETERS

Libra Enneagram 6 mermaid who loves to grow fragrant flowers near the Salish Sea. Drank for 51 years, and I now enjoy every day—just as it is. I love my sober friends and virtual tribe from around the world.

I was born in 1955 to middle class, second-generation Irish Catholics. They were part of a hearty drinking culture, fostered by their religion and post-prohibition alcohol use disorder.

In my upbringing, I assumed that alcohol in some form would be an important part of my life as a grown-up. That belief system came early, easily, and thoroughly. I also observed that drinking made things better.

As the years went on, without even realizing it, I began to gravitate toward any social function or living situation that involved drinking.

Fraternities offered free (!) beer to me—a 17-year-old freshman at the University of Washington. I don't recall how we acquired it, but we often "pre-functioned" with alcohol in our sorority rooms before we went to the dance or party, where more beer would be served. This is how I learned to drink before functions as a means to loosen up.

As a young adult learning to entertain, deciding what booze to buy for a meal was as important as what food to cook.

I believed everything the commercials said about how wine made things romantic or how beer was refreshing.

In my chosen profession (fisheries biologist), my drinking ability put me on the same level as my all-male colleagues. It was common to drink shots of whiskey after a long day of flinging 20-pound salmon around on a spawning day.

I felt my best—or so I thought—when I was shit-faced.

All my parents' friends and relatives drank. Or so I thought.

Becoming alcohol-free has turned those beliefs upside down. I've realized how narrow my life focus became by only including a life where I could drink.

I am a scientist who readily believed all the published articles regarding the health benefits of wine, yet I continued to deny that drinking every day could adversely affect my health.

In 2005, I was arrested for drunk driving. Although I had already pulled my car over to the side of the road to walk home, that didn't matter to the courts, as my key was still in the ignition and a cop had seen me drive into the parking lot. I blew .24 BAC.

After my conviction, I continued to deny that I had a problem. I ignored the proof around me by focusing on the technicality that I hadn't been driving when I was arrested.

I had a court-issued ignition interlock unit—a "blow-and-go" —installed in my car so I could not start the car with any alcohol on my breath, but I would buy mini bottles of liquor at the Quick Stop for when I got home.

I went to the required AA meetings—at least twice a week— and lied to those people about trying to get sober. I was not one of those people.

I only counted the drinks I had when I was paying attention to calories or if I had to get up early in the morning.

I'm ashamed to say that even after completing a five-year, court-approved "deferred prosecution" for driving under the influence of alcohol, I still drove after drinking until the day I quit.

Towards the end of my drinking career, loved ones, such as my husband and sister, began to offer well-intentioned suggestions that I should quit or cut back on my drinking. They believed I could moderate my drinking—only have one or two. That was impossible.

I didn't know that I could quit drinking. Honestly. I didn't think it was possible. Also, I didn't believe that I was an alcoholic because all the alcoholics died.

For 51 years, alcohol was in my system, on and off. I didn't believe or understand how much it affected me until it was gone. Now, I am amazed that I am free of it.

FREE.

I found my freedom when the COVID–19 pandemic hit, just after the publication of Laura McKowen's book *We Are the Luckiest*. She started conducting meetings in her home, and I attended. Because I was doing everything suggested to stay sober, I turned on my camera and shared frequently. I cried and shared my first year of sobriety with complete strangers almost every day.

I now openly tell anyone and everyone who will listen that I denied I had a problem with alcohol. I think getting sober is a secret superpower!

MEGHAN ROHAN

Forty-year-old mother to an incredible seven-year-old boy and a two-year-old mini golden doodle. Sober since August 2, 2020. A securities enforcement and litigation defense attorney living in New York City. Since getting sober, I have enjoyed meditation and yoga with varying levels of success. My favorite place on the planet is Central Park before 9:00 a.m. when my dog can rush off leash.

If I could give myself one piece of advice on my Day One, I would say hold on until Day Ten. On my Day One, I didn't know it was the end; I didn't want the end.

The two years before I quit drinking were very hard. Each day I focused on merely enduring my waking hours until early evening, when alcohol would mercifully ease my anxiety, loneliness, and despair. I used alcohol to hold my life together while I cared for my four-year-old son and built my career as an attorney in New York City. I knew alcohol as the portal to everything good in life—friendship, love, and relaxation.

Alcohol temporarily quieted my chaotic mind, physical pain, and self-loathing. And so, on my Day One—24 hours after I had blacked out while playing a board game at home—I didn't resolve to quit drinking for good. I resolved to keep alcohol in my life—no matter what.

I committed to seven days without alcohol, intending to prove to myself that I could go through a week without drinking. I'd hoped I would discover a newfound ability to moderate my alcohol use with ease. Deep down, I feared that alcohol had become essential. I hoped I was wrong.

I grew up in rural Vermont. During my childhood, adults routinely began drinking at five o'clock. I knew no sober adults. I do not remember thinking about alcohol as a child, except cringing when I accidentally took a sip of my father's fruit punch instead of my own. Alcohol was subtly and insidiously woven into the fabric of how my child brain understood and constructed adult life.

In high school, I drank on the weekends at friends' houses. When I was 16 years old, drinking led to a very close encounter with sexual assault. My friends and I had spent the day walking around Northampton, Massachusetts, drinking screwdrivers out of water bottles. I remember walking down the street laughing, then meeting an 18-year-old through an acquaintance.

I suddenly found myself incapacitated in a park while he caressed my face and body, with none of my friends in sight. My best friend, Lucy, who had not partaken in our screwdriver escapade, happened to drive by. She slammed on the brakes and ran over, shouting at the young man to get off me. I remember her putting her passenger seat all the way back and my crawling inside her car for the short drive to her home, where her mother lovingly cared for me all night as I threw up. I woke up the next morning hungover and humiliated. I blamed myself for my perceived failure at drinking. I vowed to stay in control, to do better.

Better never came.

In college, I started blacking out from binge drinking. The first time I blacked out, I was terrified. But by my senior year, blackouts had become routine anecdotes my friends and I joked about the following morning. I continued to binge drink in law school, but I told myself that everyone else around me did too.

I assumed that after I passed the bar exam and started practicing, my alcohol intake would naturally temper. But the stress of private practice and long hours turned drinking into a nightly routine.

Sometimes I drank two glasses of wine and went to bed. Sometimes I had two martinis and a bottle. Hangovers became an inconvenient fact of weekend life, but they rarely interfered with work. On countless Saturday mornings, I would marvel at people on the street who did not seem ill with self-inflicted alcohol poisoning, as if a life without hangovers was as much an option for me as a life without breath.

I first googled "Am I an alcoholic?" when I was 26. I wasn't looking for help, but for confirmation that I was not an alcoholic.

I knew my relationship with alcohol wasn't healthy, but I convinced myself it was normal. I saw my coworkers, professors, and peers appear to seamlessly incorporate the substance into everything that mattered: baby showers, holidays, weddings, case victory parties, and even funerals.

Alcoholics could not look like me; they weren't fit with graduate degrees and apartments in swanky Manhattan neighborhoods. My alcohol intake showed I had arrived. I binge drank at restaurants with three Michelin stars. I sipped scotch at happy hour with the white male partners at my law firm and developed (faked) a vocabulary for wine. Looking back, I can see how I felt like a fraud in my life—and how alcohol protected me from that reality.

My son arrived just after I turned 33. I hoped motherhood would magically transform me into the sophisticated, moderate drinker that I imagined I could be. It did not. I continued to black out; I continued to drink bloody Marys at 11:00 a.m. on Saturdays.

My Day One was another attempt to quiet the soft voice of the little girl inside me imploring me to stop hurting her. On Day Two, I sat next to my then-four-year-old son watching *SpongeBob SquarePants* and dug my nails into the couch. The intensity of alcohol craving leveled me. It felt intolerable.

Day Three brought the same intense, lonely craving. I could barely speak.

Day Four was no better. I endured and made it to Day Seven by immersing myself in podcasts about recovery. Something inside me cracked, and I buckled under the weight of the truth. I was addicted to alcohol, but a life without it felt like a death sentence.

Even though my experiment was meant to last only a week, something kept me from drinking on Day Eight. On Day Nine, instead of googling, "Am I an alcoholic?" I googled for help. And I found it.

Camera off, terrified and curious, I attended my first recovery meeting online. With shaking hands, I typed my day count into the chat online. And the sweet voice of Brooke Mayes, the first of many angels in my recovery, read my words out loud to a group of over 100 people. "Meghan, on Day Ten. Way to go Meghan; I am so glad you're here."

And right then another person knew; another person saw me in my discomfort. I came back the next day and the next. Recovery is an agonizing, life-giving process. It requires putting down the thing that distracts you from facing yourself, from taking responsibility.

If I could say one thing to myself on Day Ten, as I cried on the couch, exhausted and terrified, I would say "This is it, sweet girl, this is you doing it. This is what recovery looks like."

What I have learned during the last two-and-a-half years is that the magic of recovery is not in finding the right book, meditation, scented candles, or yoga practice. To me, recovery is the courage to sit right beside myself and be exactly where I am. Recovery is being here, typing this. This is doing it. This is recovering.

My advice to myself—and to you, dear reader—is to find that sweet spot inside you that comes alive with playfulness and wonder. Put down the easy button that keeps her hidden. Walk out of the dark woods and into the light. Don't hold out for the current of life to fix the thing that is hurting you. Take responsibility. You deserve it.

Two months into sobriety, my son asked me, "Mommy, why is it so fun now?"

"What, baby?" I replied.

"It," he answered.

And I knew what he meant—the being, the aliveness. A world where there isn't anything separating you from the person you love. The joy in the right now. I never knew "it" could be like this.

MEREDITH WEST

"Forty-ish year-old mother of two amazing kids, wife to the most patient man, caregiver to an angry and narcissistic elderly mom, and friend to many wonderful humans. I'm a boss lady in DC on Capitol Hill, hostess with the mostest, PTA volunteer, and exhausted woman who thought she deserved wine as a reward for doing All. The. Things. An Enneagram 2 people pleaser with too many balls in the air and suffering from massive overwhelm, quietly and slowly got sober and free on February 1, 2021. I stay sober by telling the truth, practicing daily gratitude, sharing my shame and pain with sober sisters, and putting myself first. Finally."

I never intended for my Day One to be my Day One; I just knew I needed to do something different. I knew I couldn't continue to beat up my body, to lie to my husband about my drinking, to miss my kids' childhood while in a wine-induced fog, and I was betraying myself, the version of me who had been using wine to hide, to feel less smothered by motherhood and my job, to escape from my very critical elderly mother who lives with us, to soothe my overwhelming anxiety, and to disappear while still being physically present for my family. I planned to just take a break and get my shit together.

I decided to try to make it one month without alcohol, a feat I hadn't achieved since I was pregnant with my youngest child. To be honest, I wasn't very confident that I could do it. I had failed at "Dry January," so I decided to try again in February, a shorter month. I joined a support community for moms who were doing a dry month together, and since I'm not the kind of woman who lets others down, I had to make it through those 28 days without alcohol for my new friends.

In retrospect, I wouldn't do it differently if I did have to do it all over again—which I hope I never have to do, now realizing that I can never drink alcohol. But I would have been kinder to myself on Day One. I wouldn't have spent my days and sleepless nights obsessing over all my regrets, beating myself up, and feeling deep shame around my drinking.

I made it through February 2021 and felt a little better physically, so I decided to do one more month. Just one more. Those 31 days of March felt like an eternity, but I made it. Then the moms' group I had joined, called "Dry Together," had a speaker the following weekend, and I wanted to go and be with my new friends. I couldn't drink before that, as that would betray the "dry" spirit of the group, so I ended up just deciding to do one more month.

And so it went, month after month. "Bird by bird," as Anne Lamott says. "One day at a time," as the adage goes. But sometimes, for me, it was hour by hour. Learning to cope with my emotions and stress and anxiety without the numbing relief of wine left me feeling like an exposed nerve. I experienced many ups and downs. Life didn't stop being "lifey." My anxiety didn't just magically disappear, though it diminished with the break from alcohol. And my job situation was perhaps more challenging to navigate than it had ever been. But I just kept swimming, as Dory says in *Finding Nemo*.

I had been reading all of the "quit lit," and upon finishing Laura McKowen's *We Are the Luckiest*, I joined The Luckiest Club

(TLC), her sobriety support community. As a very "all or nothing" person, I went all in. I had to. If I didn't go "all in" to meetings, I would go "all in" to wine again. My husband and children were so proud of how well I was doing, and I didn't want to let them down, so I kept going.

Discovering community was a game changer for me. For the first time, I didn't feel alone in my struggles with not only drinking, but also with motherhood, friendships, family dynamics, and diet culture.

Through TLC, I formed a little "Gratitude Circle" with three other sobriety-seeking women. We checked in with each other daily, sharing five things that we were grateful for over Marco Polo video chats or texts.

I really believe gratitude changed the wiring in my brain. Some science is behind this thought, but for me, each of those gratitudes felt better in my soul than a glass of wine. I didn't want to dim the gratitude for my son's snuggles, my daughter's laughter, my husband's steady patience, my peaceful mornings alone, or my delicious cup of dark roast pour-over coffee—for freaking wine.

While I wouldn't do my journey to sobriety any other way, because it's worked for me, I wish I had known some things on Day One to be kinder to myself:

- Alcohol is an addictive substance. Our society tells us we are supposed to drink, but not too much and not too often. It is not your fault that you have become addicted to alcohol.
- You need and deserve radical self-care. Rest, simplify your life as much as possible, ask for help, cancel anything that doesn't light you up with joy, and put yourself first for a change. No one else can do this for you, so do everything you can to give yourself the strength and headspace you need. If you have to take five bubble baths a day and go to bed at six o'clock, do that. I give you permission. Now is the time to put *you* first. You are worth it.

- Treat your own pain like you would that of your best friend. The things you've been through in your life, the trauma you've experienced, the neglect your inner child feels, is too big, too hard, to be fixed with something as simple as a drink. You deserve true relief, and alcohol won't make your pain go away. Go to therapy, do the work of healing yourself, and show compassion to your own soul for all that has happened to you.
- The anxiety/ "hangxiety" you feel on Day One won't last forever. The tight ropes around your chest will loosen, and you will start to more clearly see the subconscious ways you have been masking your true self. This "becoming" will not be easy, but you deserve to discover who you are meant to be.
- Now that you know the true impact drinking has on your life, you can't unknow it. You can't unsee it. If you start to romanticize drinking again, you know that it can never be as carefree, as satisfying, and as fun as it once was. You know too much now. You know it's keeping you from the peace and freedom you truly want.
- You don't need a "rock bottom" to stop the self-destruction. Forget the common view of alcoholics in our society—those drinking out of a paper bag under a bridge. You don't need a DUI or to lose your job or to destroy your family to stop drinking.
- Boundaries are imperative. Clear is kind. People-pleasing is dishonest. Let go of others' expectations and stop giving a fuck about what anyone else thinks of your body, the messiness of your house, your job, your parenting decisions, your quirky taste in music.
- Find community and invest in it. Support others. Help someone else though a bad day. Being a listening ear to another sober human will make you realize that you are not alone. The people in sobriety support meetings

understand you like no one else. They've been where you've been; they just get it. And you will feel stronger in your sobriety when you serve others in their sobriety.

- Poet Mary Oliver's quote, "What are you going to do with your one wild, precious life?" hits me in the stomach every time I think about drinking. On Day One I didn't want to waste my one chance at life in a fog of drunkenness. And on Day 956, I want to spend it in a fog of drunkenness even less.

- As my sober sister Whitney Bishop once said, "You still have time to create the you that you want to be." It's not too late. The world needs you to use this life you've been given for good, not waste it away by drinking.

- Just focus on hitting the pillow sober today. Don't "future trip" by worrying about tomorrow or your upcoming vacation or the next holiday. All you can control is what you are doing right now. And now. And right now.

- There is no shame. Drinking isn't a moral issue. You have used alcohol, and addictive substances to self-soothe your pain. This is not your fault. But you have better tools now, tools that will actually help you to heal.

I had to stay sober for others on Day One, but today I stay sober for myself. I am worth it, and you are, too.

SUSAN BRYANT

Retired professor of photography. Happily married 26 years. Mother of three happy adults. I'm an artist, a wife, mother, sister, friend, and TLC subgroup steward for photographers. I love to share my passion with others, and I'm always drawn to the Light.

What held me back for so long? Fear and Ego.

Fear of the idea of living a life without alcohol to calm my anxiety. (Even though I discovered—almost too late—that alcohol was fueling the fire of my anxiety.) Fear of the idea that I'd never be able to have fun at parties, at art openings, while I cooked and ate, while I made my artwork behind a camera, and in the darkroom and hand-coloring.

How did I deny I had a problem with alcohol? I was highly functional.

The side of my brain that was still defending the amount of alcohol I was consuming was my Ego (I call this particular size of my ego, my demon) saying, "You don't have a problem. Look at all that you are doing and what you have done. You can get up at 7:00 in the morning, prepare for classes, work-out at the Y (cardio and weights), teach a yoga class several times a week, and teach three photo classes each semester, along with all that's involved in academia in addition to teaching."

I had received recognition for my teaching and recognition as a local artist and founder of the first artist's co-op in our city and was a board member of our local theater in charge of the annual art auction fundraiser; I was a soccer mom photographer (and not missing a soccer game in 13 years, even though I was usually secretly drinking at the games while taking photos), maintaining an active exhibition record. I made new work, attended work-shops, entered juried exhibitions, added exhibits to my resume, had solo exhibits, and lectured about my work. I was selected for competitive artist residencies. I'm an Enneagram 7, and I have all those traits.

I had many periods of controlled drinking and abstinence. I didn't drink for two years in my mid-40s to prove to myself and my husband that I could lead an alcohol-free life. But in my heart and brain, that was not a forever commitment, just a temporary reprieve. During this time, I had two teenagers.

As I approached 65 and my retirement from my lifelong career, my anxiety increased. For one thing, the department I worked in (and my 35 years of things from my office and class-room) moved into a new building. I was thrown into planning and ordering equipment, having to take on the role of bookkeeper and technician for enlargers and cameras. During those last three years, my drinking increased, and I hid bottles in my home, purse, closet, and—something I said I'd never do—in a locked desk drawer in my school office so I could have the needed and deserved glass of wine between classes.

Alcohol began to run my life. I plotted when and where to buy it in order to have enough in stock at home; how and where to dispose of bottles; staying close to the bar at parties and receptions …

I made countless bargains with my husband and myself. I drank when he was away from home. I hid mini bottles of wine and vodka in my suitcase when we traveled. The times he found hidden bottles left me feeling so much shame but also indignation.

I thought that "I" should be in control of how much I drank, no matter what statistics and proof he told me about my drinking as a disease.

One year, about 11 years ago, I lost 50 needed pounds. To do so, I abstained from alcohol, rehired a personal trainer, and prioritized what I ate and how much I exercised. I felt good in the smaller, size six version of me. Of course, I deserved new clothes to reward myself for getting in shape. I increased my personal credit card debt with night-time, online purchasing. After only a few months, I was somehow able to bring alcohol back into my life without gaining the weight back. This was another reinforcement to my denial of alcoholism. "How bad can it be? I am back to my body from my 30s and still able to consume two bottles of wine a day or wine plus vodka," I told myself.

I began to isolate at home more toward the end—staying up later than my husband at night, so I could "prepare for my class the next day" (to drink more). I didn't have horrible hangovers. No one could tell how much I drank. Another curse, another "How bad can it be?"

I rarely acted drunk; I simply did what I needed to keep a continual buzz. That demon part of my brain would say with a singsong voice, "I'm having a party and nobody knows it." I never got a DUI. I never blacked out from alcohol.

I did not have a low bottom. My Day One was not planned. It was two months to the day after my 37th commencement, and I was preparing for an important solo exhibit of my photography to be held in the gallery of the art and design building, which would open in late August.

I had started seeing a therapist in April to help me figure out how to cope with anxiety. I lied to my therapist about how much I drank. I told her I was in charge of my drinking, and that it wasn't in control of me, but that was a lie.

Another voice in my head said, "You won't be able to afford a $500 a month dependency when your paycheck is cut tremendously. And how will you moderate when my husband goes to work and you're home all day on your own?"

So, these two parts of my brain were battling while I no longer had the ability to get off the roller coaster that was my life of drinking and secrets. Until the morning of July 1, 2019. On that morning I woke to find several empty wine and vodka bottles laid out on the guest room bed, telling me, once again, that my husband was aware of my continued "affair" with alcohol.

On that morning, when he came to me in defeated tears, I experienced a miracle, a surrender. God's voice spoke from inside me, saying "It's time. Let go. I've got you."

I felt so much fear and uncertainty, but at the same time, I felt relief and I felt as if I were being held. I promised my husband I'd go to an AA meeting, which I did. I found a sponsor and worked the steps. When COVID-19 shut things down in March 2020, I had received my eight-month chip and then miraculously discovered Laura's book, which others have mentioned, and then TLC.

I would tell my Day One self: It will be OK. *You'll* be OK. You're done. It's over. It's time to surrender and to ask for help. There will be a day (many days) in the future when you will not even think about alcohol. You will experience more freedom and joy and relief and acceptance and blessings than you can ever imagine. You are not walking (crawling) away from something, you are walking toward something: the Light, a new life, a chance to live with integrity and Grace.

TODD C. KINNEY

Todd lives in Omaha with his wife, four kids, and two wiener dogs. His passions include traveling, golf, and hanging out with his family when they let him. He invests a ridiculous amount of time and money following his beloved Iowa Hawkeyes. His day job is as a lawyer.

Fear. That's what held me back the most. I had a whole list of reasons why I shouldn't or didn't need to quit—but it all came back to fear. Fear that life without alcohol would be boring. That people would think I was weird. That I would never have fun again. That I would never get invited anywhere again.

I was afraid life would be dull. I thought I would have this perpetual nagging sadness that I had to refrain from the one activity that made everything more fun. I couldn't imagine not being annoyed or sad that I wasn't drinking. I figured (hoped!) it would wane over time, but not completely go away. Like a hole in my heart that would never quite be filled—almost like the death of a loved one. Who wants to voluntarily do something that will make them feel sad and annoyed the rest of their lives?

When you're drinking, the idea of quitting does make you sad. And when you're in the early stages of giving it up, not drinking can annoy you incredibly. It seems like everyone in the world is drinking around you—and they're loving it! They're having the best time ever! Everybody is laughing! Nobody is getting hungover or doing anything stupid! Drinking is awesome!

This annoyance seems like it will last forever. It doesn't, I promise. For me, it lasted less than a year. It was strong and ever present for about the first six months or so, then it gradually began to subside.

What flipped the switch for me was when I heard quitting described as a legitimate grieving process. You really do go through a period when you grieve the loss of your "friend." Drinking was a reliable friend that had been by my side for 25 years. It was there for everything—good times, bad times, happy times, sad times. Every momentous occasion in my life—every mundane Friday night and everything in between. You name it, alcohol was there.

So it makes sense that I grieved the loss of alcohol. Even if it had brought a lot of bad things into my life, it was still something that had "been there" for me for a long, long time. Once I looked at it through the lens of grieving, it was so much easier to understand why I felt the way I did. I was able to process my thoughts, let them work through me, and move on.

After a few months, I started to think of quitting drinking as gaining something, rather than giving something up. I had been so stuck on the idea that I was giving up this lifelong friend, this partner who had been with me forever. My whole perspective, all my thoughts, came back to the idea of giving something up. Nobody likes to give up things—especially things you like to do, or think you need. That makes us squirm. It's uncomfortable. I was so focused on giving something up that I couldn't see the possibilities for what I could be gaining.

At the time, I had no concept of everything I would gain. I couldn't possibly have known those things before I experienced them. I heard people talk about life without alcohol. I heard people say it was the best decision they had ever made. I heard people talk about how much their life had improved. But I couldn't really "get it" until I went through it myself. But it is worth it. I'm no longer annoyed or sad that I don't drink. I'm a little sad I didn't give it up sooner.

When I compare my life with alcohol to my life without alcohol, it's no contest on what I enjoy more. Life still happens, of course. Work stress, parenting obligations, relationship issues ... all of that is still there. But dealing with life is so much better. It's easier. It's lighter. It's calmer.

The best way I can sum it up is: There's more of the good stuff and less of the bad. There's more peace, less anxiety. More connection, less distance. More presence, less distraction. More self-esteem, less shame and regret. More honesty, less deception. More calm, less chaos. More feeling, less numbing. More confidence, less self-doubt. More clarity, less fogginess.

There's more gratitude—so much more gratitude. I thought I was a grateful person before I stopped drinking, but the amount of gratitude I have now doesn't even compare to before. Every facet of my life has improved. I'm more present and available for my kids. Knowing that myself, and knowing my kids also feel it is priceless.

Above all, there's more living, less escaping or just getting through the day. This experience has been amazing, invigorating, and unexpected. It's a life I never knew was out there. And it far surpasses any buzz I ever got from drinking.

If you would've told me before I quit that I would enjoy a life without alcohol this much, I would've bet you just about any amount of money that you were full of shit. I never would've believed it in a million years. I was as sure as I've been of anything that a sober existence would be more boring than when I drank.

Being so convinced of that and then discovering this whole new way of doing life that is better turns everything upside down. It makes me wonder what else is out there that I'm not even aware of right now. It's incredibly powerful to do something you once thought was impossible.

That life is out there if you want it. You don't have to experience a "sufficient" rock bottom before deciding to give up alcohol. I thought I did, and that kept me stuck for a long time. Your rock bottom can be not wanting to be hungover again. It can be not remembering a conversation with your son or daughter. It can be the shame, regret, and anxiety that comes hand in hand with drinking too much on a Friday night. It can be wanting to remove something from your life that increases the chances you will get cancer. It can be simply wanting to feel better or live a healthier life. It can be anything. Why wait for the "bad" rock bottom to happen?

On the rare occasions when I would seriously contemplate quitting, I would always remember the people who said that giving up alcohol was one of the best decisions they had ever made. Some said it saved their lives. Others talked about it like the change was a miracle.

I was skeptical at first—partly because it seemed impossible and partly because I didn't want it to be true. After I heard it from enough people though, I reluctantly started to entertain the possibility that they might have something. "Surely, they're not all in on the same lie, right?" I asked myself. Having taken the plunge and lived on the other side, I can assure you that they were not all in on the same lie.

If fear is holding you back, like it was me, I get it. I can't make that fear go away—nobody can. What I would suggest, however, is that you set that fear to the side. In its place, put all the inspiration and hope you might feel from reading this story and the others in this book. Lean on all of that for now. Borrow some faith if you have to.

Instead of letting the fear dictate your relationship with alcohol, let whatever you feel from reading these stories guide you. See where that takes you. If you can do that, I think you'll love where you end up.

Author: *I Didn't Believe It Either: My Discovery That Everything Is Better Without Alcohol*

www.toddkinney.com

ANDREA WILEY

An explorer with an insatiable sense of curiosity about myself and the world around me.

I think what has surprised me most about living an alcohol-free life is how much I have grown and evolved—and continue to do so.

I used to believe that people were set in their ways and did not have the ability to change, but now I know that is not always the case. When I made the decision to approach life in a different, healthier, more holistic way, I began to see endless possibilities for what I was capable of doing.

When I drank, I was on a never-ending loop. I would experience an intense emotion, such as anger, or overwhelm, feeling exhausted, or excited, and I would reach for a drink to lift my spirits, calm me down, or enhance my celebratory mood. I would get that instant gratification, but then I couldn't stop. I continued to drink more and more, chasing that initial buzz until I blacked or passed out. I would awaken hung over, feeling terrible, and usually not remembering most of what I had done or said the night before.

The next day I would push through my pounding headache

and nauseated stomach, feeling as though I deserved to suffer, but simultaneously believing I was fooling everyone around me into thinking I was fine.

"Look, she can do it all, she can have it all" was one of many lies I thought I was convincing people of.

Then I would repeat the cycle all over again the next night. I would drink to bring me back to "normal," then chase the chemically induced sense of buzzed relief, getting drunker and drunker, more and more obnoxious, less and less like my true self.

When I quit drinking, several months passed before I could honestly say that I felt good. I experienced glimpses of clarity, moments when I noticed that my body felt stronger and healthier, and I enjoyed nights of deep uninterrupted sleep. All those brief instances were enough to keep me going on the sober path, but a long time passed before I was aware of those experiences daily or could confidently articulate how not drinking made my life better. To this day, the hangover-less mornings never get old.

I realized early on that I needed a deeper understanding of why I drank—what I was trying to numb or run away from that was buried deep in my core. For a long time, I convinced myself that I just wanted to have a good time in fun social settings, and alcohol was a vital part of that culture.

But in reality, I wanted to escape the unaddressed pain of my childhood, the abandonment of my dad's suicide, the conditional love I received from my mother, and my feelings about myself that were the result from those experiences of unworthiness and feeling like I am "not enough."

I made those discoveries through lots of therapy, journaling, reading books, and listening to podcasts. I explored topics such as co-dependence, emotionally immature parents, internal family systems, mother hunger, and childhood trauma. My need to explore and develop grew as I discovered more and more about myself and how my early experiences shaped who I had become and how I approached everything.

Before long, I realized that I was really seeking a more mean-ingful life, but I had to understand where I came from to determine where I wanted to go. Quitting drinking was just the tipping point that let me begin the journey towards change.

I made lots of discoveries and slowly began to connect each lesson I learned along the way. I found that listening to others' stories made me feel less alone. Reaching out to trusted friends and family about my struggles enabled me to release the burden of carrying that heaviness around. I felt validated when they understood, but even when they didn't, I felt relieved to be able to speak my truth aloud. Being vulnerable with those who were willing to do the same with me opened my heart in a way that I didn't know was possible. Practicing gratitude daily let a light of positive energy in, brightened the negatively cast shadows, and illuminated my overall perspective.

I realized that the more I healed, the more others around me healed as well. I believe the more I opened up, some loved ones recognized a change in me that they wanted to experience. Whether they were conscious of it or not, they began to be more introspective, too, which also led to significant changes, like they're going to counseling for the first time, seeking out EMDR (Eye Movement Desensitization and Reprocessing therapy), setting boundaries, or trying meditation. Who knew growth and evolution could be contagious?

I've found a real sense of power in asking for help, asking for what I need—whether it is from a person or the universe. This was extremely difficult at first, but the more I requested aid, the more positive results I received, and therefore the easier reaching out became.

Accepting the things I cannot change in any given situation and recognizing that I can only control my attitude and actions gave me a new outlook on life and how I approach my daily stressors. My consistent practices of meditation, breath work, and yoga taught me how to get comfortable in stillness, feel my emotions, be present in any given moment, and listen to my heart so I could begin to follow it as a guide. Instead of not knowing what to do with peace and quiet, I actually crave it now. I can just be.

I am amazed how being open to trying one new thing leads to

another and another. It leads to exploring new topics, discovering new skills or interests, or meeting a whole new community filled with other like-minded individuals who welcome outsiders and give them an authentic sense of belonging. Ultimately, that openness continues to play a vital part in my healing.

As I heal, I understand myself more—who I truly am and what I truly want, especially after trying to please others and conform to others' expectations for so many years. Over time, I realized I had to stop waiting for someone else to give me what I need because I am the only one who can truly do that. When I love and take care of myself, I show up for others in a more present, wholehearted way. That process is the key to my never-ending growth and personal development, and none of it would be possible without my sobriety.

CATHY CHARLES

Yoga, walking in nature, writing, having live concerts in my kitchen where I am the lead singer. I've been sober for four years, mother of two kids in their 20s. I am a high school counselor and yoga and meditation instructor. I was a late-bloomer drinker, starting in my 30s. I was classy, chardonnay with *ice* always. I am a geek about science related to our bodies, specifically the nervous system. One of my trauma responses is that I do everything on my own; I do not like to ask for help. #Work in progress. According to many "loving colleagues," I can often be a yoga evangelist. According to my sister, I am an evangelist of a popular discount grocer.

What has surprised me most about an alcohol-free life?

That I eschewed alcohol for eight months with the "Cathy plan" and survived.

That once I went into community, I realized I was not alone.

That becoming sober was not about willpower.

That I never had tools.

That all of the sudden I had strengths I never knew I had.

That no one was coming to save me, but I saved myself by asking for help.

That I became a yoga teacher.

That I became a writer.

That I speak about my journey openly, out loud, and often.

That I am having a blast!

If you would have told me on July 22, 2019, I would be happy, joyous, and kicking butt four years later, I would have thought you were annoying. If you would have added that I would be a woman who is financially stable and thriving, have love of self, be a yoga instructor who founded a yoga recovery program, become an alcohol-free coach and meeting leader for Reframe App, and love to learn science, I would have told you to stop pretending I had hope. Yet here I am.

For the first eight months, I just thought I was a weak human who had no willpower. I had tried to quit drinking many times and went to therapy, but I didn't get what I needed.

I look back on it all now, and I think if I had been told, "Just keep practicing; what is your practice plan for this week?" my process of quitting would have been softer. It would not have been full of shame, self-loathing, crippling depression, and anxiety, and most of all, I wouldn't have gone into complete isolation.

I had cut back several times. Ninety days was my limit. The year before, I walked away from chardonnay with ice (because I am classy), I started to cut back. But I realize now the torture of the bandwidth I spent on thinking about it is what led me to quit.

I made a Cathy plan when I walked away. I told no one. I gave up meat, dairy, sugar, and alcohol at once, so that my mind could focus more on the other things I was giving up instead of alcohol. I refused to tell my primary physician what I was doing because I didn't want to be judged. I went to an acupuncturist (which I still do). I purposely researched a therapist who did not believe in group therapy for treating alcohol, and I started writing a gratitude list every day.

Sometimes, I think OMG how did I not drink over those eight months? Now, I know community and connection is where all the healing begins, shame melts, and strength prevails. I often say, "My drinking career ended just like how Forrest stopped running in the movie, *Forrest Gump*. He just stopped without a plan and said he wanted to go home now. That is how I feel. I put down the bottle and didn't have a plan, but I wanted to go home to me."

I have finally arrived home, comfortable in my own skin.

My greatest personal achievement in my alcohol-free life is that I am truly comfortable now with being uncomfortable. I love the adventure of it! I used to believe that brave people jumped out of planes, lived in exotic places, were yoga instructors who teach to the masses, or were soldiers who go to war. Those people were not I. But then I put down the chardonnay with ice, and slowly, I found out that I could be my own hero.

I found that I had so much time on my hands once I stopped drinking, stopped numbing. I filled it with meetings and learning more about myself by attending seminars. I had the opportunity to become good friends with many people around the world online who were like me.

Just after my second soberversary, I began to attend yoga online with a community. I found my journey to be like the alcohol-free journey. I was in physical pain with a sciatic nerve issue. I would not turn on my camera, just like when I started in the alcohol-free community. The more I practiced, the less pain I had.

I found out things like how the body holds our emotions. It all made so much sense. All the work I had done in my sobriety for two years was being let go in my mind, but my body was still holding onto it. I learned how to practice yoga poses that released pain and trauma. After a month, I started to turn my camera on, and when there were workshops, I would offer reflections.

The founder asked me after one of the classes if I had considered becoming a yoga teacher. I thought that was a hilarious question, "Me? I can't even walk!"

The founder explained that yoga was more than just the physical workout and that my life experiences and lessons were healing for others.

I got comfortable with being uncomfortable and dove headfirst into yoga teacher training. I was the oldest person by 20 years in the class and had no real yoga practice of my own. I felt so embarrassed at first. Yet, the teacher and the amazing group of women from around the world who trained with embraced all I did have to offer. I felt confidence I had never experienced in my life from being vulnerable week after week during the training. I finished my yoga teacher training on my 50th birthday and invited all my alcohol-free friends from around the world to celebrate the class with me online.

I had to select a theme for my classes, and I chose, "Grounded in Gratitude." I will be forever grateful for my sobriety. From my opportunity to lead a yoga class for those in the alcohol-free-to-cut-back world, I met the head coach of Reframe App. He invited me to become a meeting leader and a coach for Reframe App.

I now lead the age 50-plus group weekly, along with other meetings, and I individually coach those who are choosing to look at their relationship with alcohol. I love the Re"FAM" community, and it's an honor to lead people home to themselves.

Becoming sober and teaching yoga has given me a life I never would have dreamed of ever having. I fell in love with learning about how the nervous system works and how our bodies hold onto experiences. I went beyond getting certified to teach yoga. I geeked out on the mental health aspect of yoga and became certified in both trauma-informed yoga and yin yoga.

By day, I am a high school counselor. I have now brought yoga and mindfulness into my career. I teach students strategies from breathing, stretching, and how to connect their mind and body. I coach many of the athletic teams, teachers, and classes, using yoga as a mental health empowerment tool.

I am now the founder of my own yoga company, RewYre_U. My vision: mental health empowerment through all things yoga. My classes include a few different passions—one is for the alcohol-free-to-cut-back community. I created a 108-day discovery-to-recovery program.

Also, I hold classes that include a topic and share circle before practicing yoga together. This way we are practicing in a community to connect our whole selves. My other passion has been developing programs for teens through all things yoga for mental health empowerment and to walk people home to themselves who have never connected their minds and bodies as a whole. That is, for now, my greatest achievement. Every day, I just keep following the alcohol-free breadcrumbs and life keeps getting more fantastic!

"Everything in life is a practice," is now my motto. I practice sobriety, yoga, gratitude, and all things that lead me home to me daily. Most of all, I believe that community is where it all begins and ends.

www.rewyreyou.com

CHRISTOPHER

I am passionate, happily married, loyal, creative, adventurous, open-minded, loving, LGBTQIA+, and sober. I am now free from alcohol's heavy shackles and chains that bound me for years. My husband and I live happy, full, and sober lives with our dogs, since December 2020. We always marvel at how much richer and fuller life has become since we have stopped drinking. The road ahead is now bright and full of possibilities without the weight of alcohol's strong hold on my existence; it held me back from truly experiencing life and all it has to offer. My sober mind is amazing. I am *free!*

The biggest surprise I found in sobriety is *freedom* and learning that I had been a prisoner to addiction for so many years. The addiction inch wormed its way into my life and eventually took over.

Freedom, for me, only touches the surface and encompasses so many smaller and larger parts of the overall picture of what I found in sobriety. Freedom has allowed me to open up to, and enjoy, many of life's surprises—and joys it offers without my needing to be drunk, buzzed, or numbed-out to feelings.

I found that a sober life can offer so much. Now that I am

sober, I have the freedom to make decisions without having to factor in everything tied to drinking (where I can get booze and how much I should get, who else is drinking, where I can go while intoxicated and what I can do, and if I can drive). Alcohol had woven its way into every aspect of my life.

Drinking alcohol had become so normal for me that I could not see anything that seemed out of place or seemed to control me —until I did. I was shocked to find out that alcohol truly dictated almost every decision, action, and emotion in my life. Alcohol controlled what emotions I would have, how I would react to them, what I believed caused them, if I was going to hold onto them and for how long.

I was not able to understand my emotions. I was more reactive than practical with my emotions and life responses. Alcohol prevented me from attending certain events and avoiding certain activities or destinations. Alcohol controlled my time! It controlled me!

I was not living my life. I lived a life alcohol created and wanted me to live. I was not a free person to make my own decisions any longer. I was imprisoned into servitude by alcohol—to serve what alcohol wanted and created.

This did not happen overnight. The addiction snuck its way in drink by drink, slowly stole my soul, and locked me away to look from the inside at this person stumbling through life. I had disappeared. Alcohol had painted a picture in my mind that I must move through life intoxicated to feel normal.

For years I carried a sorrow I never fully understood. Alcohol preyed on this and used it to help me think I was drowning out the sadness. In reality, alcohol exacerbated the sadness.

Honesty has always been very important to me, but alcohol offered me the excuse to not be truthful, to not be me, to hide, to wear a mask, and to not speak my truth. I got to a point where I no longer drank to be social or have a good time. I drank to pull the extrovert out, to be the social guy—the one everyone wanted to talk to and be friends with.

I had painted myself into a corner or what people and I

believed I was supposed to be. I felt I had to always be the pleaser, and I lost the true me. Inside I was screaming for help, to feel happier and to be better, but I didn't know how to achieve this goal.

I got to a point where I did not know how I could possibly move through life without drinking or some form of substance inside numbing me to life. I was afraid to allow true emotions like sadness, hurt, and fears truly enter my life. I did not know how to navigate them sober. I was afraid people would not like me if I showed my sadness or made any mistakes.

Any time I fucked up or did something others did not like, I could always use alcohol as an excuse. I became a chameleon to fit in. Even at times when I did not care to fit in, I just drank more.

I thought I was in so much control during my active drinking days. After I quit drinking, I realized I was never in control at all. When I stopped drinking, my thoughts became clearer. These thoughts did not come right away, but they did slowly, one by one, find their way in. With my sober mind, I could no longer hide from my thoughts and feelings, even if they made me feel uncomfortable. I got to a point that I had to let them in. I had to learn how to welcome my emotions, feel them, understand them, and let them move past.

I have learned not to hold onto any one emotion for too long. I need to embrace them all. This has been hard, scary, and a complete challenge, for sure. So often I have wanted to just numb out and hide from them.

As I continue with my sobriety journey, I find triggers may come and go, temptations may rise, and habits are real, but I have found a strength I never knew I had. I have found I am capable of doing *me* and finding me. I don't have to live or be anyone or anything for anyone. This all came naturally once I stopped hiding and put the bottle down.

The sober me is awesome and so clear. I see that now. Why was I so scared to see me, to be me, to have an opinion? All these things that held me back from sobriety were all in my head and held no truth. The truth is, I am finding I love the newfound freedom. I now make decisions based on the situation and what I want instead of making them depend on what I think I want or what others tell me I want. I am finding a whole new kind of fun. I am finding the beauty in being able to remember what I did and be accountable. I am finding I love being able to be more present and remember my vacations or conversations. I love that I no longer have to wake up in the morning with regret of what I did or wondering why I did something outsider of my core beliefs.

I don't have all regrets from my drinking days, but I do desire to better understand how I lost control, and I never go back. My entire alcohol journey was not negative, and I have many wonderful memories that did include drinking. However, that chapter of my life is over. It went on long enough! The novelty of drinking wore off long time ago, and I missed the memo. Drinking became my church of addiction.

So, I am breaking old habits now and writing a new story as I venture on through life. My life does not require me to have a drink to experience any part of it. As a matter of fact, by not drinking, I have a much clearer head to truly experience all the beautiful things life can hold for us.

When we truly open our eyes and let life in with a clear and sober mind, the magic is endless. I now live my life sober and understand that I can drink at any time if I choose, but right now I am choosing not to and enjoy all the gems that sobriety brings.

ERIC JOHNSON

I am an adventurer, runner, certified executive coach, outdoors enthusiast, and podcast host. I am also a champion for those who are trying to recover from addiction. I'm CEO of The Luckiest Club, co-host of the *Inside Job* podcast, a certified executive coach, and a lover of the great outdoors and '90s grunge rock music.

A therapist once told me, "Sobriety is a muscle." It takes a lot of work to get into shape, and then consistent attention over time to maintain it. So, I approach sobriety just like I would any other element of my emotional or physical health—with simple, daily attention, practice, and coaching.

I describe paying attention to myself as "self-observation" because it implies both an element of curiosity and an act of attempting to learn. It's deeper than self-awareness—it's self-understanding. As nerdy as it sounds, I spend a fair amount of time each day just trying to understand how I'm doing.

For starters, every day after I wake up, I pour a cup of coffee, fill my water bottle, and sit at my table with my notes. I close my eyes and try to put words to how I feel. I try to be specific, and I write a few notes about it in my journal. I close my eyes and scan my body, noticing the aches and soreness in my joints and muscles, while also looking for any tension in my gut or shoulders —which is usually a sign that I'm stressed out about something. Then I take a few moments and scan my mind for the one or two things I am most concerned about getting to that day, and I write them down. Then I finish my coffee while watching the sunrise, or the rain fall and get ready for my run.

This whole routine takes me less than 10 minutes, but when I'm done, I feel like I am really clear about how I am showing up in my day. Clarity and direction have been the most important tools for me to get and stay sober, and they also help control my anxiety and my relationship with anger. If I get a chance to repeat this again in the late afternoon I do, but doing this every morning is non-negotiable.

Non-negotiables are a core part of the second element of staying sober for me—practice. A series of rituals that I follow throughout the day keep me grounded and sober. Some of these are directly related to sobriety and others focus on helping me feel like I'm living a good life and taking care of myself. The most important thing I have learned about non-negotiables and daily practices is that fewer is always better! Sobriety doesn't have to be complicated!

My first daily practice is to run every morning. I run outside, even in the rain, unless the circumstances are extreme. I run without headphones so I can be fully present in nature, aware of my surroundings, and mindful of my body and breathing. Moving, sweating, and being outdoors are critical practices to my sobriety—they control my anxiety, build my stamina, and increase my mental resilience.

My second daily practice is to drink 90 ounces of water. I fill a bottle in the morning and refill it twice throughout the day. Feeling hydrated helps me feel healthy, and it also keeps me from feeling thirsty in the late afternoon, which can lead to cravings.

My third practice is journaling. I don't sit down and write everything all at once; I write in two- to five-minute increments throughout my day as I engage in self-observation. I find it's easier to stick with in short bursts, and I get more out of writing when I feel strong emotions.

My last practice is engaging my mind through reading and music. When I have something to pay attention to, I am so much better at managing my mood and how I'm stimulated externally. I read a page every day in *The Daily Stoic,* and I usually try to read for at least 10 minutes before bed. I rotate between fiction and non-fiction—and I have no problems steering away from "quit lit" and memoirs. In early sobriety, it was helpful to hear the stories of others, but now that I am approaching 10 years of recovery, I just read whatever I find interesting.

Music has been my absolute savior. I play records in the background all day, as it sets a great mood for me, helps me keep my groove going, and provides an outlet for some fun. More acutely, a song exists for every mood, so if I feel a triggering emotion, such as sadness or anger, I have something I can turn to that helps me sit with the feelings until they pass. I can honestly say that if it weren't for Pearl Jam and the Foo Fighters, this sobriety thing might not have stuck for me!

My final element of sobriety is coaching. Despite having nearly a decade of sobriety, and being the CEO of a sobriety support organization, I have no delusions that I know everything, am prepared for everything, or am immune to my demons. I talk with a therapist every other week, and I am completely honest with her —I chose one who calls me on my bullshit so I can't talk my way out of my problems. She makes me face them head on, and that has been the only way I've been able to overcome the challenges that life has thrown my way.

I also attend sobriety support meetings nearly every day, and at minimum, five times a week. To be clear, I lead sobriety support meetings, but I don't count those for me. I go to meetings as an attendee to listen, to support, and to share. In early sobriety, I thought a day would arrive when I didn't have to go to meetings anymore. But because sobriety is a muscle, and because being part of a supportive community is a gift, I want to go to meetings almost every day. Hearing other people talk about sobriety gives me new ideas, fills me with compassion, and creates meaningful connections. All of this is critical to my getting and staying sober.

So that's how I do sobriety—through daily attention, practice, and coaching. While it may seem like a lot, it isn't. But more importantly, the reward of a good and healthy life makes any and all work worth it.

STEPHANIE HERNANDEZ

Avid reader and lover of all things made with plastic building blocks. Mother of two goldendoodle good boys. Finding my true authentic self—one sober day at a time.

I don't mean to sound like a broken record, but I've just kept it simple, even when it was the most difficult.

I'd had five months of sobriety in 2021, and most of those five months were spent floating on a pink cloud. I didn't have to practice most of the tools that were presented in meetings, because the joy of being sober and remaining sober kept me trucking.

As soon as that joy dissipated, I was back to drinking and ignoring everything I had learned in my meetings. I am grateful for that pink cloud. It taught me that joy was possible, and it kept me safe from facing the very hard things until I was ready for them.

I didn't know my last drink would be my last. I was drinking in secret, and not a lot of people knew about my relapse. It seemed to work for me. I would stay sober for about a month and then have two to three nights of heavy drinking. Then it was back to repairing my body for a few weeks.

I was anxious and angry and lashing out at those closest to me.

I didn't know how I would ever stop again—it felt truly impossible, even though I had stopped once before for five months. Then one day, about a year later, I signed into a meeting, and I saw the beautiful souls who supported me through my first round. I was just as happy to see the smiling faces and welcoming smiles as they were to see me. I was overwhelmed with love and gratitude and I didn't know I truly needed that until later.

I didn't decide to stop that day. But that day I did decide that I needed support. I realized that how I was living wasn't working for me anymore.

Those five months of clarity opened so many doors for me, and I had just changed my career and had a supportive boyfriend. Why was I unhappy? My body urged me to make a change. Was only drinking a few nights a month actually working for me?

I didn't decide 21 days in, when I was asked to be part of this book project and said yes. I didn't decide two weeks in, when I called an "old timer" who had been sober for decades. I was trying the things people had recommended. I was taking it one day at a time.

I decided this time I would listen to the people who helped me through my first time and accept them as human beings behind the small squares that appeared on my laptop. I started actually connecting with other sober people.

Today, I accept that I am exactly where I need to be, and when things get "drinkey" for me (a term I use when I consider turning to alcohol again), I go down the list of my tools. I share it out loud. I text and call my sober friends. Not all of my tools work all the time, but I know where to turn to when I need extra support. My tools sometimes included such things as getting into the bathtub at 11:30 p.m. until the alcohol sales stopped at midnight.

I am 228 days sober today, and I am finally learning what it means to take it a day at a time. My journey has been such a work in progress. It is proving to be more difficult to confront the things I was trying to numb myself from. I am learning to be gentle when those drinkey thoughts come up. I followed those impulses for so long, and of course my brain is wired to go that route. I accept the thoughts and go down my list of tools. Why do I want to feel different right now? Why am I craving to change the way I feel and escape?

My life isn't perfect, as I thought it would be at almost eight months sober. I thought I would have a perfect job and lose 20 pounds by now (at least). I thought for sure, by now, I would qualify for the Boston Marathon and run a Fortune 500 company. My wins come to me in small and digestible moments that have not much to do with any superficial and vain accomplishments. Qualifying for the Boston Marathon would be great, but what about those small moments on Sunday mornings when I remember everything I did the night before? Those small, powerful moments show up for me when I least expect it. Kind of like my sobriety, it is here and I accept it. I accept that what I am doing is the work. My work started long ago when I started to accept that I needed help. It started the day I asked for help.

My life just simply is lifey. I am present for it when it's hard and present for it when it is easy and joyful. I have met fabulous friends on my journey, and people who live healthy lifestyles have surprisingly gravitated to me. I continue to connect. I will continue to fail at lifey things and have moments of panic where I think I will not make it through—but I do.

Not alone though, I have those who understand this struggle and support me. The valuable thing I have learned is that I don't know everything, and it is okay to ask for help. I am being patient because I know this work never stops. Even though it doesn't always seem like it's worth it, it always is. Don't ever give up.

RORY FLANIGAN

Artist/fashion designer residing in the Pacific Northwest. Goth-chic. Flower-obsessed. Drinking was robbing me of precious time to love, create, and nurture.

I have always been slightly obsessed with the idea of *Memento mori*. As a fine arts undergrad in art history class, discovering the concept that symbolism in art has served as a reminder of our mortality for centuries greatly appealed to my dark (morbid?) romantic sensibilities.

The words are Latin for "remember that you die," and memento mori is a style used in classical still life paintings known as *vanitas*— skulls arranged with flowers, fruit, candles, books, hourglasses, and timepieces as well as other objects that possess an oblique reference to impermanence.

The imagery—a moment in time—is meant to remind us of the ephemeral nature of life. The flowers will die or are already withering, the fruit will rot, and the candles are waxy stubs in their sticks or have just guttered out—imparting a curt trail of feathery smoke.

The skull, inanimate and bereft, is jarring amongst the assortments. Skulls are placed on books—whole or sans jaw—on their sides or staring blankly off canvas. They are bleak among sexy, corpulent tulips and bright embryos of pomegranate seeds. The brittle bone contrasts starkly against the creamy skin of juicy apricots. They are in the shadows of refracted light radiating from beveled crystal goblets and gleaming pocket watches. The lonely skull is relegated to prop status and minus life, a shell.

The idea of contemplating my own mortality was not entirely new to me since I attended Catholic school from age six and Mass since I could walk. "Rory, remember that you are dust, and unto dust you shall return," Father said solemnly as he traced a cross in thick ashes on my forehead—ashes that would get caught in my eyelashes and would eventually work into my eyes for an irritating afternoon in class.

This early introduction to the concept of my own impermanence was made particularly personal by the priest's substitution of my first name instead of the customary, "Man."

As a young person, the reminder of death or the idea that my mortal body of me would someday be ashes was morbidly interesting but was so abstract it was irrelevant. As taken as I was with memento mori as an artistic or literary trope, it was relegated to the academic or artistic (or decorative) parts of my world.

I loved skull imagery and reading the stoics and other writers of classical antiquity who espoused and practiced philosophical memento mori. The ancient Roman poet Horace is credited for writing the oft-appropriated *Carpe Diem,* "Seize the day!" as well as another more obscure phrase: *Nunc est Bibendum,* "Now is the time to drink!"

Along with my artistic and other liberal arts pursuits, I also loved to party. I would *carpe* that *diem* all night long and justify it by recalling biblical or literary memento mori "eat drink and be merry for tomorrow we die" (Ecclesiastes 2) or drinking "life to the lees" (literally), as Lord Alfred Tennyson encouraged. I was young. I devoured life. I lived to be high on alcohol and drugs— the exhilaration and the freedom of being in an altered state.

The early days were so bright. They glittered with spectacular promise. I was young, beautiful, and felt immortal. Entire nights and into the next day were spent reveling in the laser-sliced fog of nightclubs or in churning derelict warehouses. The sun would come up and I would marvel at my world, the beauty of the sunrise and hundreds (sometimes thousands) of young people pulsing with music and life. It was life in technicolor. I never wanted it to end. I truly believed that I had found a way to tap into the essence of life—I had become part of a collective beauty. It felt otherworldly. I felt I mocked Death with my voracious living. I was "sucking out the marrow of life" as Thoreau so carnivorously desired.

Then, slowly, a tinge of sadness greyed the edges of my life. A loneliness seeped into me, and I could not drink or party it away. A denser, more sinister chill took hold, and I could not shake it. I was terrified by this darkness. Everything was bleak and contaminated. I was in shadows. I could hardly eat. I felt desiccated, hollowed, and cold.

It took years for me to feel warm with life again. I grew older, and while the electricity (and resultant depression) of the early days was not as intense, I still drank nearly every day. I still sought that brightness and camaraderie in happy-hour hedonism and after-hours bars. I enjoyed being very drunk. I loved the alternate reality. It was my favorite place to be.

I still admired memento mori and believed I was honoring this message by partying well into my 40s and by "celebrating" with daily bottles of wine. I routinely purchased the most expensive champagne that I (really couldn't) afford. It was time to toast to life! Even if it was Tuesday during the workweek. My sentiments were always noble—however, like my appreciation of memento mori, a bit misguided.

I did not have one rock bottom—rather I dragged myself across rocks intermittently for nearly 30 years until I had the (literally) sobering realization that my life was pretty much half over. How much of my life had I wasted by being wasted?

Suddenly my beloved memento mori took on new meaning. Was I willing to waste more of life impaired, incoherent, blacked out, or hungover before I joined my bony brethren? Maybe "seizing the day" didn't equate to binge drinking or a cocaine-bender. Indeed, I would spend the next day horrifically hungover in bed, with depression and crippling anxiety as companions.

It took me a few years (and many Day Ones) from those realizations to fully abandon drinking. Towards the end, I employed forms of memento mori to cancel the madness. The still lifes, skulls, and the haunting words of the stoics inspired me. I downloaded an app that pushed quotes about death by poets, philosophers, and celebrated thinkers. "Remember you are going to die" pops up on my home screen five times a day "at random times, and at any moment, just like death," as the developers explained.

Desperate, I wrote sticky notes reminding myself what I sacrifice or might lose when I drink and stuck them in various places— in drawers, on bathroom mirrors, and inside cabinets. Two and a half years sober, I still find them. Contemplating death is my daily habit, much like meditating or writing a gratitude list.

Considering death is a powerful reminder that life has an expiration date. I have found this to be motivating in all areas of my life—not just in maintaining sobriety. I am no longer willing to sacrifice my "one wild and precious life" (thanks, Mary Oliver) to alcohol, drugs, trivial matters, toxic people, hangovers, or soul-stealing jobs.

By sitting with death, I honor life. I have given myself the gift of the present moment—and it's there that I found the wisdom, beauty, and the infinite youth that I had been seeking.

CARLY SCHWARTZ

Carly is a writer and tech executive based in San Francisco, California. She has founded media organizations in San Francisco, led newsrooms in New York City, worked on financial inclusion initiatives in Mexico, and built a journalism school in the Panamanian jungle. She is currently leading content strategy at Google's moonshot division, earning her master's degree in narrative therapy, and finishing her first book—a memoir about recovering from addiction and depression while living in a 15-person commune. Her two greatest loves are traveling and spending time with her Boston terrier, Nacho, but unfortunately those two activities don't often go hand in hand. She's a former total party girl who went on weekend-long benders and drank mezcal straight from the bottle.

It's noon on a Sunday, and like most Sundays, I'm still in bed. I woke up three hours ago, that adrenaline-fueled, sleep-deprived jolt that happens after a night of tweaky tossing and turning. I'd shuffled downstairs, head pounding, and smeared some nut butter on an apple. I ate it standing up. Chugged a mason jar full of water. Beelined back upstairs before any chance encounters with my roommates. My heart still racing from the night before, I nosedived back into my bed, smashed my face into my pillow, and tried to turn my body off once more.

But now it's noon, and I still can't relax. The idea of doing anything productive makes me anxious—three weeks' worth of laundry is heaped on my sofa. The idea of doing anything active makes me nauseated—my mind is speedy, and my limbs are dizzy. The idea of doing anything social makes me want to hide under the covers for the rest of the year. I only want one thing, and I want it now: whip-its.

The smoke shop is only a block and a half away, but I might as well be summiting Kilimanjaro. It's one of those postcard-perfect 68-degree early afternoons, and around me, couples stroll hand in hand, licking ice cream cones. Teenage girls hoist shopping bags over their shoulders from the vintage clothing store. The coffee shop teems with hipsters, and the line at the bakery is as long as it always is. People living their lives—not a hangover in sight, unless they're really good fakers.

And me, laser-focused on my destination and the reward awaiting me when I reach the peak of this concrete mountain.

My heart pounds faster as the cashier rings me up. *What's taking so long?* I can already taste the nitrous in my lungs, that sweet, sparkly release. I can hear the *pop* of the canister and feel its icy exterior. I'm just going to do one or two and then get to my chores. I'm lighter-footed on my walk home; the sun is still too bright, but my headache is gone.

I leap back into bed and inhale my first one. Two at a time is always better. May as well. Before I know it, 15 empty canisters are lined up by my side, a neat little row. Then 20.

Do I even like this feeling? What's so special about this three-second release? I can barely feel a thing. One by one, I twist and suck, telling myself each time that this one will be my last. But now I've reached the bottom of the box, and I may as well finish it. An entire carton of whip-its, gone in less than 20 minutes. Guilty and foggy, I grab a garbage bag and sweep the empty canisters inside. They make a jangling sound as they hit the floor. I get back into bed, even more anxious than when I first woke up, and stay there, in and out of shallow sleep for the next four hours.

I've been struggling with major depression for the better part of two years. Sometimes the depression is the paralyzing kind, which makes it impossible to get out of bed, which makes walking down the street feel like trudging through molasses, which makes everything from taking a shower to writing an email feel like an insurmountable chore.

Other times I describe it as "walking depression." I'm highly functional, making it into the office, charming coworkers during meetings, even gathering with friends for drinks after work. But I can't turn off the negative thoughts or endless loop of self-loathing in my head, whether I'm laughing at a party or curled up in the fetal position for the 16th straight hour. It's excruciating. From time to time I think about ending it all; once, that notion grew so powerful that I wound up in the hospital.

Lately I've described my depression as a tale of two Carlys. There's the Carly in her default life, and she's pretty depressed. Getting up is nearly impossible; most days, I send half-conscious emails from my bed until at least noon. One time I even gave a remote presentation to a group of 50 coworkers slumped across my pillows, the video function on my Google Hangouts turned off because of a "slow connection."

Every once in a while, I cancel all my meetings and sleep all day, rising groggily around sunset to pick up a salad around the corner, which I eat with my roommates, dodging questions of "How was your day?" I refuse to meditate or cook or exercise. I've lost interest in everyday activities I used to love, like listening to music and reading magazines and taking bike rides.

Then there's Party Carly. Party Carly uses her social life as a distraction from depression. When I'm not in bed or procrastinating, I'm with my friends. Being extroverted lets me forget about the lackluster state of my life. When I'm socializing, I can ignore my problems.

And that social life, more often than not, involves substances. I knock back a drink or five at the wine bar after work. I run around parties with a bottle of mezcal in my hand, pouring it into people's mouths. I naughtily suggest whip-its on a Wednesday. And every two weeks or so, I'll go on a cocaine bender that lasts 12 hours, hoovering white powder up my nose like there's no tomorrow, feeling like the belle of the ball. Being on coke is the only time I experience mania, the antithesis of crippling depression.

It's safe to say that these days, when I'm happy, I'm high.

The problem with Party Carly is that she makes regular old, depressed Carly feel a whole lot worse. The lows get lower. After a bender weekend, sometimes I stay in bed for two days or more. After a three-day cocaine binge this summer that took me from Mexico to Los Angeles, I got into bed for a week, emerging only for a boozy dinner with a friend. The next day, I was on a flight to London, where I spent several days; each day I slept until noon and stayed out until sunrise.

But that recent Sunday afternoon with the whip-its felt different. I felt out of control. I sucked them down so quickly that it terrified me. I didn't know what the long-term bodily consequences might be or whether my behavior would negate the effects of my anti-depressants. I decided to do something I knew I should have done a long time ago but had deliberately avoided: I shared every detail of my substance use with my therapist.

When my therapist first suggested treatment, I thought she was overreacting. I told her I sometimes went weeks without even drinking and reminded her of the two months I spent sober last fall.

She explained that a common misconception of addiction is that to be an addict, you have to use every day. She asked if I honestly thought I could give up my party weekends on my own (I couldn't). She said my refusal to exercise or engage in any self-soothing extracurricular activities suggested that I wouldn't be able to integrate sobriety meetings into my regular schedule (I wouldn't). What I needed, she suggested, was a full-life intervention—an intervention that would not only arm me with skills and coping tools but would also force me out of bed every day, at a regular time, and into a healthy routine I could carry back into the real world.

My psychiatrist was even more adamant. My brain may need up to a year to recover from my cocaine use, she told me. And inhaling nitrous oxide was especially problematic—I could cause irreversible brain damage.

Rehab felt like a realistic next step.

So here I am. Some of my friends have laughed this decision off and told me I'm overreacting or that I just want a vacation. They don't see me in my lowest moments, alone in my room. They know me as a mischievous party girl with a dark side that's sometimes hard to control, yet never impossible to reign in. And I haven't lost everything: I still have a good job, a respectable bank account, close relationships.

But I need help. I deserve to know what it's like to experience happiness without a bottle in my hand or a baggie in my pocket. I deserve to have a reason to get out of bed that doesn't involve a party. I deserve to walk down the block on a Sunday afternoon and smile, not because I'm on my way to buy drugs, but because the sun is shining.

I deserve to know what it feels like to live.

DEBBIE ADAMS

Mountain momma to boys. Lover of pets. Voracious reader. Outdoor adventurer and stargazer. Pursuer of wisdom, joy, and rest. Awakened to the beauty of life since 2020.

Rock bottom. The words bring terrifying images to those of us outside of recovery. Swirling pictures fill my head—homeless, destitute, alone, nothing left to lose. These images were fed to me by a society that kept telling me that as long as I drank responsibly, I wouldn't end up there. That those types of things happened to hobos and drunks, not respectable people like me.

Rock bottom was for people who didn't have any will power or control. So, where was I when I hit my rock bottom? Was it as dramatic as that? Had I lost my job, was I living out of my car, drinking wine out of a paper bag?

No, yet I was just as out of control, lost, and terrified. I was ashamed, riddled with guilt, and confused on how I had ended up here.

On September 15th, 2020, I awoke on the couch. I was not sure what time or day it was. *Are the kids in bed? Is it morning? Why am I on the couch? What happened?*

I was groggy, confused, and not sure what was going on. I struggled to reorient myself. *What the hell happened?*

I found my phone. 8:45 p.m. The kids were fine; they are downstairs playing on electronics. What happened? I fell asleep. I was just so tired. Life had been so hard with the separation, trying to figure out where I stood, what I was doing with my life, how I could support the kids and myself.

Yet, I know I didn't "fall asleep." I don't fall asleep while the kids are awake. I passed out.

I stumbled to my feet and felt so much disgrace and shame. *Who am I? What am I doing? How long will this go on? Is this the person I am, the mother I am?*

For so long, I had told myself I drank because my marriage was in shambles. We didn't communicate, I didn't want to be in the relationship, I was lonely and sad, and yet, there I was. Now the marriage was over, and I was passed out on the couch after drinking three-plus bottles of wine at 6:30. *What the actual fuck?*

I got up and tried to get a handle on the situation. *I need to get the kids to bed.* I was having a hard time; I felt awful and my head spun. I was so tired and dehydrated. I was shaky from not putting anything into my body besides nicotine and wine.

I just wanted to crawl back into bed, yet I knew what I need to do.

I had little patience for my kids' needs, and just keep shouting that they needed to go to bed. I begged them. "Mom just doesn't feel well. Please, just go to bed, so mom can lay down."

I was irritable, harsh, and simply not a good mother. I hated to be this kind of mother.

I can't think about that right now, I just need to get them to bed so I can go back to sleep.

I finally accomplished this after much yelling and crying. My nervous system was shot. But all the emotion and adrenaline pushed me past the edge of sleep. I huddled in bed, weeping, wondering, how I got there. Pleading with myself, God, anything, to help me be done with this. Making the same promises I made a million times and feeling how hollow the words felt. Fearing I would break my heart again tomorrow, not believing I was enough to make this change. Terrified that tomorrow evening I would be lying in this same bed with these crushing feelings of shame, guilt, and despair.

How do I move forward? How do I leave alcohol behind?

For years, I had known I had a drinking problem, I remember calling AA one night and praying that there was a meeting at 3 a.m.— and angry when there wasn't. I knew when morning came, I would rationalize or normalize my drinking.

I kept trying to figure out a way to keep drinking because I couldn't understand a life without alcohol. It seemed unfathomable. How would I get through—the idea made my blood run cold and my heartbeat fast.

How would I manage life without alcohol? I took it everywhere I went—in the car, in my purse, to the kids' t-ball games, to pumpkin patches, everywhere. There wasn't a place in my life where alcohol wasn't allowed. It was what I did, it was how I made it through the day.

The idea of life without a drink seemed impossible; not only impossible, but empty and void of joy. I was looking for the elusive third door Laura McKowen so aptly describes—trying to find the middle path, instead of choosing the path of alcohol or sobriety. I didn't want to continue in this way, but I didn't want to quit alcohol. I wanted the door that would let me drink normally again, because if I couldn't drink like that again, then what was the point? I would never have fun and feel comfortable again; my life was over—with or without alcohol—and that was the most heartbreakingly depressive realization.

My Day One was like so many of the other Day Ones I've had. My latest attempt at getting sober had been going on for about nine months, and I rarely could get past a week. I felt so weak and helpless, each day swearing to be done, and yet, each day picking up again. And now with COVID–19, I was starting to drink earlier and earlier in the morning.

Yet, something was shifting. I had started reading quit lit. I had signed up for a 90-day challenge with OYNB (One Year No

Beer). I had reset my challenge many times, yet each time I found the people were supportive. They offered me grace and kindness and told me I could do the same for myself.

The idea of self-love was a foreign concept to me, but slowly it started to sink in. I began to fathom the idea that beating myself up would not get me sober. If that worked, I would have been sober years earlier. I realized that only by being kind and accepting of myself would I find the strength to get sober. I needed to believe that I was worthy of a big, beautiful life. Heck, I just needed to believe I was worthy of a life.

Slowly I created a new life. I saw how I could implement small changes that would help me get healthier. I couldn't tackle everything at once, but slowly I was learning new ways of being, thinking, and understanding the addiction of alcohol.

The books, *Alcohol Explained* and *This Naked Mind*, profoundly affected me. They helped me to see that alcohol was an actual poison, that I had become addicted to an addictive substance. Alcohol is meant to be addictive, and the reason I couldn't quit it was not because I was weak or lacked will power, but because my body was physically and mentally hooked.

A light bulb illuminated in my brain, and my sobriety journey was forever changed.

What was different this time? On that September 15? I can't honestly tell you. It was the coming together of all the knowledge I had obtained over the years of wanting to quit drinking. It included the kindness and compassion I found in the sobriety community, the brilliant words I had read, and the touching memoirs that also told my story.

You cannot unknow the truth. I knew I deserved more, that my kids deserved more, and that this life had more to offer than hangovers, guilt, and shame. I finally realized that I was worthy, and that I just had to quit for now.

As Laura McKowen describes in her book, *We are the Luckiest*, I didn't have to do forever, just for now, and again. I learned I just needed to begin again each day. And for now, not to drink—even for just this one moment, and then again.

That morning I woke up and made a video to remind me of how bad I felt and why I didn't want to do this anymore. The last thing I said on the video was, "and remember Debbie, you are worth it."

That is how I overcame my rock bottom and found my last Day One.

HILARY BOYCE

I am a foodie, occasional retreat chef, server, coffee connoisseur, quit lit book junkie, Enneagram 2, half-assed runner with very little yoga. I am a divorced mom to two amazing kids who are 18 and 19. I have been sober since January 23, 2016, and it was the worst thing turned to best thing ever! I live to help other women get over "mommy wine-drinking culture" and the shame that creates! I am passionate about gathering around the table and connecting people through good food and stories.

I certainly had given up any hope of getting sober. I had reached a point of deciding, "I guess this is who I am and what I do."

One morning in mid-January 2016, I looked at myself in the bathroom mirror unable to recognize who was behind those eyes. I woke up yet another morning without a hangover, because when you drank as I drank, with a steady IV drip-line style, it no longer bore any ill effect.

Occasionally I would get the shakes and require a gnarly grease bomb breakfast fast food sandwich to get my day going, but mostly I was a professional blackout drinker. Close to 42 years old, a shell of my former self, a hollow human being existing with one aim: to fulfill my insatiable thirst.

My world had grown so small. I had children in fifth and seventh grade and no longer was allowed to pick them up from school as it was assumed I would be buzzed/incapacitated before their school pick-up time of 3 p.m.—and that assumption was not wrong. The most tragic part of the last days of my drinking was how much my drinking schedule controlled me. I had waited seven years after marriage to have kids and considered being a mom the best role of my life. Yet now I wasn't even showing up even though I was so driven by a relentless obsession to one day drink normal amounts.

My drinking had started at age 27 as an occasional glass of wine at the theatre or concert venue out with friends or when I was hosting fun moms' nights. But my reality at age 41 included a pre-shift Fireball shot from the corner store on the way to my lunch server position, followed by a few beers in the afternoon after my shift. I would drop by the fancy bars in my neighborhood on the way home. I could no longer pick up my kids from school. I then would get home, pop the prosecco or cheap white wine, and start cooking dinner—along with downing a few bottles to pass out by midnight.

Friday, January 22, 2016, started like most days described above—Fireball shot, work, beers at restaurant alone, and headed home. My then-husband was coaching that night, and my daughter decided she wanted me to drop her at the game. I had to prove I could transport her by using my keychain Breathalyzer to show I was able to, but sadly I knew how to cheat the keychain.

I dropped my daughter off at the game and wandered in the gym, feeling like an alien around a place that had previously felt like home. I had been a coach's wife for many seasons, but this night the chasm was unsurmountable. I no longer belonged. Off I went to a brewery far from my house. That was the beginning of many decisions I would make in the next 24 hours that would alter my future forever.

A few weeks before, I'd met a guy at the bar, and on this night, I met him again for a couple of IPAs. I did the date in a brownout and managed to not let on how drunk I was when all of a sudden,

I blinked, and it was after 11 p.m. I said goodbye, left the brewery and thought I'd better take the back roads, so I didn't have to navigate the speed of the freeway. I made it from the neighboring town I was in back to my hometown.

I thought, *I'll just pop into the fancy bar in my city for last call.*

A fountain was in the center of the road, with a four-way stop. I rounded the corner and parked in front of my favorite coffee shop and across from the bar. I looked up, and flashing, bright lights were behind me. I thought I would flash my license and registration and be good to go. But when I opened my window, I'm sure ethanol punched the officer in the face—the aroma of all the pounded drinks throughout the day emanating from my pores.

"We just want to make sure you can safely drive this vehicle," the officer said. "Can you step out of the car, ma'am? How many?"

"Two, officer."

"Can you walk down the street, say the alphabet backwards…"

I miserably failed the field sobriety test in front of the local coffee shop, God, and everybody at the bar. I was handcuffed and put in the back of the car, with my Tahoe impounded. We stopped at a nearby police station before heading to the county jail.

I recall talking on the phone to a lawyer who suggested I blow —I originally thought I shouldn't, as I would sober up soon. I finally agreed and blew a 2.8. The officer looked at me like, "Only two, huh?"

We drove the 20 minutes north to the county jail, and I was starting to grasp my dire straits. I was taken in and handed jail scrubs, while they packed up all my personal belongings. They were concerned I might have wicked withdrawals, so they tried to get me to drink juice. I waited on a bench and then in a holding cell for what seemed like forever, freezing.

Finally, it was my turn to be processed. The officer quipped, "A few too many at moms' night out?"

I was finally processed around 4 a.m. The female officer had mercy and asked if I wanted a cell to myself. I said yes. I was also told in the morning that the cell would unlock for a short time, and I could use the phone on wall to call bail bonds.

I was curled up on fetal position in a cold jail cell with a paper-thin blanket. I was finally stopped dead in my tracks. I had very little left—no marriage, no home, no relationship with my children, no dignity.

I had been lying to myself and chasing the elusive, "cunning, baffling, powerful" drink.

I prayed the most honest and sincere prayer that night that I'd uttered in a long time. It essentially was, "Fuck off, God. I don't think even you can get or keep me sober, but if you do, I will do whatever it takes."

I was in the darkest spot of my life and still had the audacity to be defiant and challenge God.

The following evening, I was finally let out on bail. I finagled my last acquaintance who was speaking to me to lend me the money. The next crucial decision was whether to go right or left. Right would mean continuing the incomprehensible demoralization and walk into the many bars lined down Hewitt Ave. The county jail sat on the locally famous bar row.

Left meant to walk away from alcohol. Terrified and not knowing how I could possibly stop, I went left. I found a taxi at the gas station with a curmudgeonly driver who let me use his flip phone to call the impound company. The owner clarified that he accepted cash only, and not a penny short. I took $300 from our joint savings. I got to the shop and was $15 short—I had to literally run down the street in the dark night to the closest ATM. The next decision: box wine or Gatorade?

Gatorade and $20 cash out. I ran back, paid the strict dude, got my car, and drove home. No one was there, and I hadn't been missed. Eventually my daughter and her dad walked in, assuming I had been out drinking as usual, not coming home. I laid on my bed.

I woke the next morning and left for my son's fifth-grade basketball game, coffee in hand with all the other moms from school who were watching their sons play—yet everything was different. I was in a catatonic state, going through the motions. I couldn't pull off the illusion that everything was okay.

That night I met with an attorney. He laid out my options: A<B<C< D. I had another decision to make.

For a split second, my mind told me that maybe I could pay a lot of money get out of it. But I knew that if I did, in only a matter of time, I'd get a second DUI, and I'd be back again because the root of my problem. My soul would not get the help I needed to live if I tried to cover it up.

I could finally get rigorously honest. I chose Option D: Deferred prosecution.

JAMIE ARMSTRONG

I am a retired Fire Captain/EMT. Married 40-plus years. Father of four, grandfather of four. Friend of dog, Grendel.

During dinner last Sunday, my brother turned to me and asked, "What was the rock bottom moment that made you stop drinking?"

This was unusual. I love my brother David dearly, and we've had dinner together every Sunday night since the death of my mother two years earlier. Just the two of us—my wife had given up on our silliness. David and I had established a Sunday routine. I would prepare a nice meal, after which we would enjoy a film noir. At dinner, we would discuss the week's events and our siblings.

His question flustered me. We had always endorsed the family tradition of ignoring the elephant in the room. Rather than holding to the clan family motto: *Invictus Maneo*, which means, "I Remain Unvanquished," our family motto should have been: *Omnia Sunt Bona*: "Everything Is Fine." My brother and I rarely discussed deeply personal issues, let alone addiction.

I, of course, deflected the question with, "It's complicated. I just stopped."

That ended the subject, and Dave and I were soon watching *Sunset Boulevard* for the tenth time.

Yet, his question stayed with me. Had I faced a rock bottom moment?

Did I experience an epiphany? Did an event inspire me to change my life?

I am 63 years old. I do not think I have ever experienced transcendence. I am not sure inspiration or epiphanies exist. My experience is that change is gradual. The effect alcohol had on my life was gradual.

Early on, I learned that alcohol was related to adulthood, relaxation, and reward. When my father arrived home from work in the early evening, the first thing he would do was to fix a drink. He would loosen his tie and make an old fashioned, Manhattan, or martini. I associated this ritual with being an adult. When I was twelve, my father once let me have some of his beer in my glass. I remember feeling grown-up.

When I entered high school, I began to drink on weekends. Alcohol made me feel less anxious and more self-assured. I enjoyed drinking, and beer was easy to get. The drinking age was eighteen, and alcohol was everywhere.

In my sophomore year of high school, my father became ill with cancer and died. My mother was consumed by his illness, and I took full advantage of the lack of supervision. I never drank during the week, but every weekend I did.

Shortly after my father's death, in my junior year of high school, we moved across the country. I became isolated from my friends and family in the Midwest. I continued to drink on the weekends. Drinking became a part of my identity. Alcohol was always there, but not yet a priority. I used drinking to become closer to my new friends. Drinking with them became a shared experience and a shared adventure. I became one of the party kids at my high school.

Upon graduation, I moved into my own apartment and began college. My college years were marked by a new independence and an increase in binge drinking. At 20, I fell in love and married. At

32, I had a newborn and a two-year-old. Several years later we adopted two more children. My binge drinking continued.

My career was as a Firefighter/EMT. I loved the comradeship of working on a team and embraced it. The firefighting culture was then, and still is, dominated by men. My shift mates became my closest friends. We worked together and lived together.

Alcohol was a key factor in our bonding. I believed drinking together with my fellow firefighters created an intimacy that I had never shared with other men. I remember believing that I had found the path to becoming a man. Together, we dealt with challenges and tragedies, and we had a reason to drink.

I easily justified my drinking. Anyone would drink if they had experienced what we had. We did not talk about our shared trauma; we buried it. The worse the call, the more we drank. Only my fellow firefighters could understand. People who did not understand were wimps. I loved drinking, and to my great regret, I endorsed and encouraged these beliefs.

I was a firefighter for 35 years. The last three years before my retirement, I had started drinking on my way home from work. Then I began to drink nightly. I started to drink vodka and hide the bottles from my wife. I drank alone.

When I retired, my drinking increased, as the guardrails of my career disappeared. My firefighter friends had no idea I had a drinking problem. With my retirement, I lost my firefighter friends. The intimate friendships that I believed in had been false, created by and reinforced by our shared interest in getting drunk.

My drinking had been progressive—slowly over the years, it had become a priority. In an attempt to control my addiction, I created rules. Never drink before five, never drink more than three drinks, only four drinks, only five drinks, never drink at or before work, only have one bottle at home.

I tried to change what I drank from vodka to whiskey because I hated whiskey. Only beer, only wine, only on Friday, only on Saturday, only on Friday and Saturday. I had to change liquor stores, afraid that the clerks would recognize me. I would drive to different towns to buy vodka in an attempt to hide my drinking. I lied repeatedly to my wife. I hid full and empty bottles all over the house. I was aware I had a problem, but I felt helpless. I was in darkness and alone.

Rock bottom—the absolute lowest or worst point.

Had I reached my lowest point? No. I used the concept of the alcoholic reaching rock bottom to continue to drink. Rock bottom? Hell! I had never gotten a DUI. I had never lost my job. I had never even been asked about my drinking at work. I had never crashed my car. I had never gone to jail.

In my mind, I had a long way to go before I reached rock bottom. Therefore, I could continue to drink.

Did I experience an epiphany, a transcendence, or an inspiration to stop? No. The world I had created through my drinking had slowly become small and limited. My life revolved around alcohol—how much I had, where I obtained it, how I obtained it, how much I drank, when I drank, and who was aware of it. I felt confined to the darkness, controlled, and limited by my addiction. I was tired of it. It was all too much.

The desire for sobriety, like my addiction, was gradual. It began as a whisper. The whisper was, "Change." I began to listen. I began to see. Then, I began to believe. Change was possible.

For me, true change did not happen quickly. I found a community. Through daily virtual meetings, I became part of an online, worldwide community. The Luckiest Club has helped me change my life and attain sobriety.

The desire for sobriety and the act of sobriety requires humility and work. Change does not begin with reaching rock bottom, inspiration, or epiphany. True change is built on the foundation of a whisper and the commitment of self-work. I am awake. I am free. *Omnia Sunt Bona.*

JENNIFER MICEK

I'm a ballet instructor and owner of the Dance Conservatory of Denver, and I love living an alcohol-free life in beautiful Colorado. I quit drinking on January 7th, 2021, in an attempt to save my marriage and I ended up saving myself instead.

Choosing to quit drinking was one of the hardest decisions I've ever made in my life. I knew that alcohol was no longer serving me and that it was holding me back from being truly happy in my life. Although I didn't have what some would call a true "rock bottom" and I was considered "high functioning" by my friends and family, alcohol was holding me back from living my best life. I couldn't figure out why I was so unhappy and trying to moderate my nightly wine habit was making me crazy. I'd gotten to the point where I could white-knuckle through the week only to drink too much on the weekends and spent every Sunday hungover. It was affecting all of my relationships, with my now ex-husband, my 3 children, and my ballet students because I knew I wasn't my best self. Because I'm a perfectionist and extreme people-pleaser, I didn't let anyone know about my internal struggle with alcohol and how much space it took up in my mind. Every morning I would wake up and think, "What day is it? Is a drinking day or not?" And if it was a weekday, my mind would find an excuse to be able to drink; it was a hard day at work, something annoying happened, etc. Finally, after a HORRIBLE hangover on Christmas Day 2020, I decided to try 30 days of sobriety in January 2021. I didn't reach out to anyone about my plan, I wasn't sure if I could do it, and because I didn't talk about it, I didn't have any support from my family and friends when I quit. No one really thought I had a problem because my life hadn't fallen apart, and I had been able to keep up the façade that everything was "fine" for years.

After white-knuckling sobriety on my own without support for almost six months, I finally realized that I couldn't do it on my own. I reached out to the one person I knew who was sober. I am forever grateful that she recommended "The Luckiest Club," an online support community where I finally found the support I needed with people who understand not only how hard it is to quit drinking in today's society, but also to be surrounded by people who wanted to see me succeed and who would listen and hold space for me as I shared my deepest feelings and emotions.

I needed connection, and I think the best thing a family member or friend can do to support a loved one in recovery is to really connect with them, whether that is through attending support group meetings with them, group therapy, or just having regular, open conversations with a lot of listening. I also highly recommend to anyone who is sober-curious, or who wants to support a loved one in recovery, reading *This Naked Mind* by Annie Grace, *We are the Luckiest*, and *Push Off from Here* by Laura McKowen (who founded The Luckiest Club online support group) and following the *Home* podcast with Laura McKowen and Holly Whitaker, which was extremely helpful to me in early recovery. Learning about addiction, the brain, and behavior helped me understand the science behind why it's so hard to quit drinking, and finding a therapist to uncover the reasons I was numbing my emotions has helped to keep me sober. I realize it's uncomfortable to talk to a friend or family member about their addiction, but simply asking how someone is doing or if there is anything they can do to help, goes a long way. Being dismissive is not the same as being supportive, and it's incredibly eye-opening to see who stands by your side when you quit drinking. There is a grieving process that goes along with how relationships change in recovery. Some relationships change for the better and some fade into the past. Learning to stay in the present will be a lifelong challenge that I work on daily with yoga, meditation, and regular support group meetings.

I enjoy thinking about ways loved ones could support someone in recovery from alcohol abuse or any kind of substance use disorder, because of my own experience and the lack of support I felt from family and friends. My life emptied out when I quit drinking, and I couldn't do a lot of things when I first quit, simply because being around alcohol made me want to drink. I had to stop going to parties, BBQs, vacations, and holidays that centered around alcohol in the first year. It would have been beyond helpful to have family and friends that came up with other things to do that didn't center around drinking, but for me, that didn't happen.

I think the most helpful thing a loved one can do to support someone is to talk and listen openly without trying to "fix" the person, to plan fun things to do together that do not include alcohol, and to ask simple questions, like, "How are you doing" and "How can I help you?" Just being there to listen and to give love and affection, and to not offer advice or solutions is helpful. It's hard to navigate strong emotions in early sobriety without the numbing effects of alcohol. It takes time and patience to "recover" who you are without drinking, especially in today's society.

Two and a half years later, I'm still surprised how my life emptied when I quit drinking. My marriage completely fell apart when I quit, and my then-husband didn't. Friends stopped inviting me to things, and although I now understand the confusion of whether or not to invite someone when it's a drinking event, I think it's better to send the invitation and let the person decide whether or not they can attend. During the first year of sobriety, it was really hard for me to attend events that revolved around alcohol, but now, after almost two and half years, it's not an issue for me anymore. It's taken a lot of work, time and therapy to get to that point, but I'm happy to be on the other side.

Quitting drinking includes a grieving process. While it's not the same as losing a family member, there is grief when giving up alcohol or any kind of addictive substance that has become a habit, especially when it involves your primary relationships. Loving, open and honest communication from family and friends can make something that is really hard turn into a relationship that is really meaningful and beautiful instead. I am so grateful to be on this path of recovering the truest, most authentic version of myself and to be able to share a part of my story to help others.

KATE MACKENZIE

Kate Mackenzie has been Sober since September 27, 2019. A mental health counselor in training. Lover of running and Barry's Bootcamp classes. I used to drink to dissociate from my childhood trauma but—spoiler alert—that was a terrible plan!

By the time I was 18 years old, I had lived through a lot of harrowing experiences. My parents went through a contentious divorce when I was six years old. My father remarried, and I gained a new stepbrother, stepsister, and stepmother by the time I was 10.

My dad was found guilty of three real estate-related felonies, for which he was supposed to go to jail, when I was 12. He avoided being incarcerated only because he was diagnosed with cancer. My father survived his first battle with cancer, but when I was 17, I learned that he had a physical altercation with my stepbrother and was admitted to the psych ward.

My stepmother divorced my dad after this incident. I did not have an opportunity to say goodbye to my stepfamily, and I never saw them again. My father remarried and divorced three times after his relationship with my mother, and he battled cancer twice before he passed away in 2012.

This lovely laundry list of trauma is the shortened version of what transpired in my colorful childhood. I never got to be care-free when I was young because I was dealing with problems that are typically reserved for adults. These experiences impacted me detrimentally because they took place during the most critical time for a human's brain development.

My childhood was riddled with Adverse Childhood Experi-ences, also known as ACEs. The more ACEs an individual experi-ences, the higher the likelihood that he or she will experience lifelong mental and physical ramifications. The odds were stacked against me in the first half of my life, but in my adulthood, I have worked hard to create an entirely different way of being.

Living through all these events as a child caused me to grapple with anxiety, depression, and CPTSD as an adult. In my life today, I participate in talk therapy and EMDR. I also take anti-anxiety medication in order to address my mental health struggles. When I started drinking as a teenager, I was drawn to the relief alcohol gave me from my pain.

When I was younger, I thought my destiny on this earth was to deal with extremely traumatic events on a never-ending loop. I suffered a lot throughout my life because of the consequences of other people's actions. I became conditioned to chaos that was the norm for my family.

Drinking became the source of discord in my life when I no longer lived with my family of origin. Getting drunk, acting errati-cally, and then feeling regret mimicked the dysfunctional cycles I had become accustomed to as a kid. I honestly didn't know how to live a stable life completely free from problems.

Luckily, a light bulb went off in my head when I was still an active drinker. I had a moment of clarity when I thought about all of the time and effort I put into going to therapy, taking medicine, eating healthily, exercising, and meditating. I saw that I negated all of my positive intentions when I drank.

I experienced an increase in my anxiety and depression every single time I imbibed. I felt worse mentally and physically the day after I drank, regardless of the quantity. Drinking alcohol was terrible for me, and it was preventing me from healing from the hurts of my past.

Many years I would progress in my attempts to grow and strengthen my mental dexterity. Then I would drink and fall backward into a pool of negativity. When I decided to stop drinking for good, my daily patterns changed significantly because I was no longer the person who was hindering my own evolution. I have been able to make significant strides in therapy now that I am clear-headed all of the time.

The coping mechanisms that helped me navigate my childhood were compartmentalizing and dissociating from my pain. At the age of six, I didn't cry when my parents told me they were divorcing. I didn't shed a single tear at the age of 12 when I found out my father had cancer. I started experimenting with alcohol at age 14. I quickly became someone who blacked out regularly, embarrassed myself often, and cried seemingly without reason. Everything I could not deal with when I was conscious, seeped out of my pores when I drank. I couldn't contain the turmoil inside of me once alcohol was part of the equation.

I continued to drink problematically off and on until I was 40 years old. Now that I have been sober for three and a half years, I can actually sit with difficult feelings. I can face things now that used to terrify me. I used to think if I even glimpsed at my childhood trauma, it would break me. I thought if I let myself cry over what I went through, I might weep forever. I thought if I allowed myself to remember all that had transpired, I would have a mental breakdown.

The good news is that I was wrong. The truth is that if I would ever get to a better place with my grief, I needed to process my trauma instead of denying it ever happened. I would never heal my attachment and relational wounds if I didn't accept the abuse and neglect that I witnessed and endured. I had to stop drinking before I started the process of accepting who I was.

In my personal relationships, I have been prone to excessive people-pleasing tendencies. I thought I had to completely abandon myself and be someone without needs in order for people to like me. These are two extremely common characteristics of codependency. Now that I am sober, I have more honest relationships. If someone hurts me, I talk to him or her about it directly, as opposed to repressing my feelings—which explode later.

I am much clearer on what I will tolerate, and I don't pretend things are okay when they aren't anymore. I haven't morphed into a perfect human being who navigates life flawlessly simply become I am sober, though. That's not feasible! I have made changes that have improved my life exponentially though. I am confident in myself now that I have made it to the other side of my darkest times. My overall temperament is a lot more even-keeled. I don't feel anxiety and depression on the same level since I stopped drinking, and the symptoms of CPTSD have lessened as well.

I feel healthier and happier than ever now that I no longer drink. Giving up alcohol is the greatest gift I have ever given myself. I feel as though I gave myself an opportunity to end the dysfunctional part of my life and start over with a clean slate.

The only regret that I have regarding my sobriety is that I didn't do it sooner.

MARK NOVIK

Divorced dad to two preteen girls. Alcohol and weed were my daily necessity for decades until I was diagnosed with pancreatitis on February 1, 2021. I have now been ready and eager to live every day. TLC, yoga, meetings, and reflection now fuel my life of *discovery.*

The best decision I ever made is my proudest of accomplishment. That decision was breaking free from alcohol and finding the courage to be me.

My last Day One from alcohol was 648+ days ago on February 1, 2021. I am forever grateful that day chose me. It took the most painful experience I've ever felt to be able to finally embrace sobriety. Today I live free from the chains that held me back for a long time.

I spent many decades wandering and lost. I started using alcohol and marijuana when I was a senior in high school. I quickly realized I could escape my feelings and troubles by numbing out and often blacking out.

I flunked out of my first year of college because I found that I preferred partying any and every day of the week to going to class. I came home and found jobs while trying to go back to community college several times over the next few years, but always dropping out. I had no direction and no purpose; I was just existing.

In my early 20s I drank when going out with friends, but I did not drink alone yet. I often smoked marijuana alone, though. I enjoyed forgetting about the world for a while and never having to pay attention to my feelings of loneliness. My relationships never went very deep because I was never living in truth. During those earlier years, I often hid my marijuana use because I felt immense shame over it.

I met a woman when I was 25, and we dated. We drank together, but she did not consume any other substances. Over that time, I hid cocaine and ecstasy use. She found out about the cocaine use when I told her I was several thousand dollars in debt. My relationship with her was built on lies; I was always trying to cover my tracks and conceal my substance abuse and the money I spent on it.

After five years, we got married and moved 1,000 miles away from my family. I felt extreme loneliness after the move. I found a job working in the evening and getting home at 11 p.m. when she was usually asleep. That's when I started drinking alone, in 2008.

At first, I didn't try to hide it much. She saw me buy cases of wine and beer. We moved into a house in 2009 and for a year or two, a neighbor would often come over at 11:30 p.m., when I got home from work, and we drank whiskey and smoked weed together until 2 a.m. He moved in 2011.

In 2011 we also had our first daughter, but lost and buried her twin brother, who died a day after they were born. We had our second daughter in 2012, and shortly after that I started buying pain pills from another neighbor. I drank alone in my basement at night and got high every day on pills and weed.

My wife finally found out about the pills in 2015, when I stole money from her and my children to pay our mortgage. I was caught and felt alone and backed into a corner, so I enrolled in an Intensive Outpatient Program (IOP) and started attending Narcotics Anonymous (NA) meetings. I managed to get 100 days clean and sober in the fall of 2015, but I was never doing it for myself, and I was not ready to find the truth.

I would get so frustrated in meetings when I didn't think I could grasp the program, so I bought beer after the meetings and drank it on the way home. I started drinking alone after work again in my basement. My wife found out about the drinking and kicked me out of the house right after New Year's Day 2017. I moved into the cheapest and smallest apartment I could find.

Now that I was truly alone, I could drink and smoke the way I thought I wanted to! I started filling the apartment with empty beer bottles, then switched to wine and finally to whiskey. After a friend I had met in NA committed suicide in the summer of 2017, I pledged to get clean again. I got almost two months and was sober for a trip to Los Angeles for my cousin's wedding.

When I came home from that trip I started drinking and smoking again, and that started to most depressive phase of my life. I was drinking 12 to18 beers a night. Then it became two to three bottles of wine. Then it became a fifth of whiskey with sugary citrus soda.

I fell deeper into a self-loathing, self-hating hole that I could see I was not going to climb out of. My wife finally filed for divorce, and we signed papers in November 2018. I had done nothing to get help and find a healthy way to live, so she legally ended our marriage, though I had checked out of it many years before that.

I moved into a house in 2019 and continued to drink and smoke and watched my physical health deteriorate significantly over the next two years. By the fall of 2020, I would get drunk and high after work every night and end up in tears in the bathroom screaming at the mirror. "Why can't you stop? What's wrong with you? You suck, and you're a loser!"

I would pour my whiskey and tell myself; *Tonight, will be different; I can stop when I want.*

But I could not stop and was too ashamed to ask for help or let anyone know what was going on. I hated myself and what I had become. I was lonely, alone, scared of the truth, my body was starting to fail, and I was ready to die. I didn't want to live in the pain and shame anymore. My asthma was out of control, and I struggled to breathe despite many meds. My blood pressure was very high. I was 5'9 and weighed 235 pounds and had become pre-diabetic while eating fast food daily. Cholesterol and triglycerides were way too high. My acid reflux was out of control.

I could not start another Day One of trying to live sober because I knew I could not do it alone, and I felt too much shame to ask for help.

On January 31, 2021, my old neighbor came over and we drank and smoked like always. I ate fast food, like I always did. I didn't know that would be the last day alcohol and fast food entered my mouth.

The next day, at 9:45 p.m., I started feeling ill at work, right before my shift was over. I was sweating, nauseated, and had new pain in my abdomen.

I told my boss I was leaving early and ran to my car. I got home about 10:15 and puked. Then the pain got very bad, very fast. My abdomen and chest felt as if they were on fire. I thought I was having a heart attack and called 911.

By 11:30 p.m., an ambulance was dashing me to the emergency room. At 2:30 a.m., after a CT scan, I was in excruciating pain as the doctor told me they found acute pancreatitis, ascites, and a very swollen liver. I looked at her and said, "I know why I'm sick; it's because I drink."

I spent four days in the hospital on IV pain meds and fluids. For two days I could barely move. I was in so much pain and swollen. I finally had nothing left to do but look in the mirror and evaluate my life. I told myself on Day Two that if I survived, I would find a new way to live. I didn't know how it would work, but I didn't want alcohol to be a part of my life anymore.

I came home from the hospital, and I believe a miracle happened to me while I was lying in that bed in pain. I lost the desire to pour alcohol and fast food down my throat. I also lost the compulsion to smoke marijuana. I started to rapidly lose weight. My body had been retaining so much fluid from my liver struggling that when I suddenly stopped drinking, I lost a pound a day. In two months, I'd lost about 45 pounds.

I went through withdrawals for two weeks and sweated profusely, and still had immense abdominal pain. I went back to work after two and a half weeks and finally got my strength back after almost a month.

I reached out to an old friend who I knew was sober and asked her how she did it. She pointed me to a Facebook group called "We Are The Luckiest with Laura McKowen" and from there, I found the online sober community called "The Luckiest Club" or TLC.

Joining TLC and finding a community that accepted me exactly as I was turned out to be what I'd always been chasing. I told my story in meetings and made friends with like-minded, sober people.

I started eating a mostly plant-based diet, and my blood and health got better quickly. I stopped taking all medications within weeks of being hospitalized. I lost about 60 pounds, and all my numbers are within a healthy range today. I love myself and I am not afraid of living anymore.

I stopped using THC on October 10, 2021, and have been free from all substances for over a year now. I thought I could not stop. I'm so grateful I did. It was the best decision I ever made—to stop fighting myself and the world.

MORGANN MITCHELL

Sober for 6.5 years. Single mama of a two-year-old girl. Fan of volleyball, baseball, hiking, running after a toddler. I'm a creative writer, a personal support worker, and a hairstylist. My drinking nickname was Captain Morgan, and everyone knew there was alcohol in my cup. If the event didn't have alcohol, I brought it. If alcohol wasn't allowed, I didn't go. There's nothing I won't go through; I'll feel all the feels. I have a hard time asking for help; don't want to be a bother. Survivor of sexual, physical, verbal, emotional abuse, childhood trauma survivor. Enthusiasts of finding the miracles in the mundane, I never say no to helping people, always up for playing with anyone, any age, anything. Gemini, Enneagram #2w1

I should just kill myself tonight.

That was the solution I came up with to deal with all my life's problems. Death would stop the pain. It would stop my problem with drinking. It would stop the destruction. It would stop the loneliness. This was my rock bottom.

This happened on January 20th, 2017, and on this night, I took my last drink of alcohol. That last drink occurred when I ran back into the house and dropped my bag I had just packed to go to rehab for three months. I grabbed a bottle of tequila and chugged half the bottle. I felt as if I were breaking up with the love of my life and ending the relationship with my best friend forever.

I was saying goodbye forever, and I was so scared. Alcohol was my everything, and then it became the thing that wanted me dead. I was 30 years old, divorced, close to losing my job for calling in so many sick days (hungover). I felt tortured by the memories of my childhood trauma trying to surface. I was trying to drown those memories by drinking, but the pain always found a way to swim to the top.

I didn't know how to feel, how to process emotions. I thought my feelings would kill me if I felt them, so I drank at them. And it worked for 15 years until it didn't and killing myself was the answer.

After a full day of drinking, like most other days, and sending out text messages to random guys to try and fuck the pain away, I was going to pull the bendy dryer tubes off, duct tape them to the exhaust of my Jeep, and go to sleep forever. I didn't really want to die; I just wanted the pain to end. That's what I really wanted to kill in me.

Something incredible happened that night. I feel like the little girl in me, the little girl whose innocence was taken from her and lived a tough, trauma-filled life … that little girl wanted to keep me alive.

So, for the first time in my life, I asked for help. I called my brother. I was full of rage. He saw past that and knew this was a desperate cry for help. He Googled treatment centers and took me to detox that night. Maybe the little boy in him saw that little scared girl in me, and for a moment we were just a couple kids trying to save a life.

I'm grateful for that moment. I'm grateful for it all—even the pain, which I now know how to feel, how to process. The pain did not—will not—kill me. My trauma did not make me strong or tough through processing it. It made me soft and gentle. It made me kind, and compassionate and empathic.

Once I stopped poisoning myself with alcohol, I became my

most authentic self. I took all the masks off that I felt I needed to feel safe in this world. I am the most *me* I have ever been.

I still get scared, and I believe in just doing things while scared. I don't wait for the fear to pass because it doesn't. While I was so scared that night of my last drink, I didn't know the miracles that would come from living an alcohol-free life.

Those miracles include living as my true self as a queer woman. I'm a single mom to a wonderful and wild two-year-old who I get to respectfully parent every day. It's been an honor to watch her grow up and let her feel her feelings—all of them. And in that process, I heal my little me too! Every time she cries, and I say to her, "You are allowed to cry and feel everything you're feeling," little me says, "Thank you. This is how it should have been. I am safe to feel now, too."

That's the best gift that living an alcohol-free life has given me, the ability to feel everything without numbing any of it. I want all the feelings forever.

I'm a good friend who knows how to show up and support and hold space (the only way I knew how to before was with a bottle to get shit-faced). Now I'm a container of love. I can pour you a glass of love—no shitty hangover included!

I never knew that I'd come to love putting on comfy pants at 7:30 p.m. on a Friday evening and staying home. I love home. I love saying "no" to things that no longer serve my soul. I no longer people-please or say "yes" to things I don't actually want to do. I now love reaching out and including people. I know I can't do this alone, and I don't want to. I'm kind, and that is my fucking super-power. I am love, I am light, and this is a beautiful life.

PAMELA NELSON

Registered nurse for 30 years. Lover of dogs and horses. Favorite pastime— listening to neo-classical piano music. Breast cancer survivor. Love to ride my bike in the woods. Libra—strive for balance. Hard time saying "no," and keeping boundaries. No one knew I had an alcohol problem. Divorced two times, no children. Sober since January 1, 2021.

"No, my rock bottom did not dictate my decision to get sober."

It was quite the opposite. I was jailed and got a DUI, but these events did not affect my drinking. My Day One really did *find me;* I did not elect it purposefully.

In the book, *Mother Hunger,* Kelly McDaniel reports that half the population has an imperfect attachment style. I realized I am among that half. I have an insecure attachment style.

On September 27, 1959, I was the first born of five girls. My dad was a Filipino physician and my mom a Caucasian German woman. My parents got married because my mother was pregnant with me. I was raised in Rochester, Minnesota. My mother always said she never loved my dad, but she had four additional daughters after I was born.

In McDaniel's book, she said insecurely attached babies carry internal distress and grow up to have an entirely different nervous system than securely attached infants, whose mothers were good at nurturing, protection, provision, and guidance.

Dad worked a lot, and my mother was a stay-at-home mom. She did her best to raise five girls, but truthfully, we were emotionally neglected with little nurture or direction. She also physically neglected us. I remember we never had to brush our teeth and often went to bed with bubble gum in our mouth—and woke up with it in our long dark hair. Mom would cut out the gum with scissors. When we went to the dentist, we had many cavities.

It was a good thing my dad was a financial provider because my mom was a spender. She never taught us to save money, she never said she loved us, and she rarely cooked meals. We had take-out fast food a lot.

Mom's main thing in life was to smoke cigarettes, drink soda, play tennis with the wives of physicians, and play bridge. Neither of my parents drank alcohol. We did have a cleaning lady, an ironing service, and babysitters often, as my parents were active in bowling, tennis, and golf.

To give my dad credit, he did insist that we all get college degrees and that we play tennis every day. I played tennis since the age of 13 and played competitive tennis in high school and in college. Living in Minnesota, we could play tennis every day because we were members of an indoor tennis club. All five of us girls were straight-A students in high school and college.

I recall first drinking alcohol when I was in junior high, and I got kicked out of a dance for being drunk. I felt lost most of my life, feeling like the odd one out. I learned in the *Mother Hunger* book that insecure attachment can show up as depression or addictions, among other things. Insecure attachment feels like, "hunger for belonging, for affection, and for security." Insecurely attached adults often struggle with loneliness. My high school and college days were fraught with trying to feel as if I belonged someplace. I also had various boyfriends throughout this period.

In high school, I did not drink much. However, I did have a serious boyfriend and, unfortunately, got pregnant in 10th grade

—and my parents insisted that I have an abortion. To this day, I lament doing that, as I always wanted to have children but was never able to get pregnant again. I did not end up with that boy, but I always had a boyfriend from that time on. I was trying to end the craving for someone or something to end the pain of isolation and loneliness and my need for affection. I think the lack of nurture, lack of hugging, and the fact my parents never said "I love you" perpetuated my feeling of being unlovable.

I now realize I have a huge hole or wound in the center of my being that longs for belonging, love, and being valued. I have spent my entire life looking to fill this hole unsuccessfully—mostly through romantic relationships and alcohol.

I finished high school with honors and ended up bouncing around between five different colleges. Eventually I earned two bachelor's degrees—my most recent one in nursing. I have been a registered nurse for over 30 years. It has been a good occupation for me.

When I was in college at Mankato State, I met my first husband at age 22. I married him because I wanted to have children. We divorced after three years of being childless. I met husband number two in 1988 and was with him for 10.5 years. We also were unsuccessful at having kids together. Both marriages were not happy places for me, and I ended up divorced twice.

In reviewing my past, it would appear I started problem drinking in 2004 when I started working in pharmaceutical sales. When I ask myself why I drank, the answer in part is that I was very sorrowful about not being able to have children.

I continued to drink throughout my pharmaceutical sales rep position into early January 2009. That industry is full of alcohol!

At one point during that time, I got a DUI while driving my company car, but because I performed well in my sales career, instead of firing me, my supervisor went to bat for me. He flew in from another state to get my car out of the impound lot and let me work with a workers' permit to drive a company car.

You might assume this incident was a rock bottom for me, but no—I continued drinking throughout my pharmaceutical career. I remember being hungover at meetings and sometimes passing out on my yoga mat before bed.

Most would consider another incident from 2008 a rock-bottom event. I was horseback riding with a friend and drinking beer. I must have gotten quite intoxicated because at one point, a park ranger told my friend and me to stop riding where we were and go to a different area.

I was flippant and uncooperative, so he asked me to get off my horse and walk closer to him. I refused, so he came toward me, pushed me to the ground, put my face into the dirt, and hand-cuffed me. He put me in his squad car, and I was yelling the whole time. As I was in his squad car, I tried to kick out the windows. Then he stopped his vehicle and put a three-foot pole device with shackles on my ankles so I could not kick any more.

This was a very shameful moment for me and should have been a rock bottom—but it did not suppress my drinking at all. I even had to spend the night in jail and have my boyfriend come and pick me up, which was very embarrassing.

In 2009, the company decreased the sales force, and I was laid off.

In my next job, at an outpatient treatment center (of all places), I was asked to leave due to drinking. The following job in 2011 was part time. I remember drinking while on the job, but I did not get fired.

Then In 2012, I started a new job and that is the year I went to inpatient treatment voluntarily and drank less but was not completely sober. Since 2012, I have not had any legal consequences because of drinking. At that time, I drank two to four beers a day, held a decent job, and did well.

In 2016, I was diagnosed with stage two breast cancer. I underwent a mastectomy and had 25 sessions of radiation. This changed my life forever, and since then, I have suffered moderate/severe neuropathic chest pain. That is the type of pain that feels like a warm iron is sitting inside of your chest, burning you from the inside out. I have been on non-narcotic pain meds ever since.

In 2020 I decided to try sobriety after one of my coworkers told me she was "worried" about me. I am not sure why she said this, but we worked closely together, and maybe she noticed my hangovers. In 2020, I also had three periods of continuous sobriety: one month, two months, and about three months.

I relapsed for a bit and started "dry January" on January 1, 2021, and have been sober since.

I attribute my success to many things: In my early days, I did a 30-day online challenge, did a Craig Beck online workshop, listened to the book *Cold Turkey* by Mishka Shubaly, and read the books *The Unexpected Joy of Being Sober* by Catherine Gray, Amy Dresner's book, *My Fair Junkie, Quit like a Woman* by Holly Whittaker, and *We Are the Luckiest* by Laura McKowen.

I also wanted to share some of the tricks that helped me be successful in sobriety:

- Playing the tape forward
- Book ending
- Doing the next right thing
- Playing effective music to help manage anxiety
- To manage cravings. When I was having severe cravings, I drove to the liquor store, and while sitting in the parking lot debating about going in, I put on a session from Craig Beck that I had saved on my phone. He talked about making a recording of how I was feeling at this moment, why I wanted to drink, and my intentions and actions were going to be—and then playing the recording back to myself until the craving left.
- Using NA beer: I drank bloody Mary mix and NA beer every day for months, then graduated to kombucha, and now drink just flavored water or juices.
- Having support. In the early days, I did five meetings a day.
- Having support through tough times. When my boyfriend of six years ended the relationship, my friend

called me and as I was bawling my eyes out. She kept saying, "Loss is hard." Over and over. This helped.

- Another tough time was when my horse died. She was *special*—the longest-term relationship I had ever had. I saw her every weekend for 16 years. She was always something I could care about and provide for and love. I had to put her down due to old age on June 19, 2021. I had support from the TLC community as I shared about this loss on group. Two plants were delivered to my home from TLC subgroups. This meant so much to me, and it was so cool that my two worlds collided—the online world and real life— receiving these two beautiful plants at my home that I could touch and water.
- Having a phone counter app. I use the app called "I am Sober."

DAVID M.

I live to interact with my kids and my wife. I've been on my journey for several years now. I remember my first sober app, my first sobriety podcast, my first TLC meeting, and my first session at Lionrock. I'm a father, husband, mentor, cancer physician, and researcher. My drinking nickname: probably "asshole" but that dates back to my years in a fraternity. I would more frequently misuse the phrase "death before dishonor" and then dishonor my body, my mind, my spirit. I'll try anything twice. I have a hard time asking for help—shame and guilt prevented me from finding community, grace, hope, and resilience much earlier. Enthusiast of vast skies and lands. No one I know likes hotter hot sauce than I do. Dare you.

Community has allowed me to give myself grace and has probably saved my marriage, my family, and my career.

I began this journey with years of pathologic drinking in my family. Alcohol became a tool to numb us from life stressors and the daily adulting ennui of dinner, dishes, laundry, etc.—all necessary, all dull.

My wife and I were using alcohol as evening entertainment, as a substitute for friendship and intimacy. We were drifting apart, and my world was getting darker. I was drinking most nights—knew it was too much but didn't address it. I keep some bourbon in the liquor cabinet and some hidden in the basement to make the liquor cabinet supply last longer.

When I went to bed, I would fall asleep immediately, but sleep was not restful, and evening conversations would be forgotten the next day. This was such a problem in my relationship with my wife that I would try not to speak or have a meaningful conversation after I started to drink, for fear of not remembering it the next day.

My father and I were very close; he was I the man respected most in the world and wanted to become. He lived his retirement quietly serving others—growing, washing, bagging hundreds of pounds of food from his garden and giving it to the food pantry in his community. He helped found a homeless shelter, ran a church free store, and supplied school children with backpacks, school supplies, new underwear, and warm winter clothes. He was at the forefront of Thanksgiving and Christmas dinners for his community. He was loving and kind and adored my children.

On a Friday in April 2019, I received a call that my father was down, and the paramedics were working on him. He had been watching TV with my mother, went downstairs, and never came back up. He was dead before I answered my phone. Probably cardiac. Just like his father. Probably how I will die as well.

So, add to pathologic drinking anger over loss, unmitigated grief, untreated depression to a pandemic, social isolation, virtual schooling, children swallowed by screens, a severe knee injury, a broken arm, surgery, months of crutches and rehabilitation, and you have a recipe for a rock bottom.

This is when I found community. Once I acknowledged that drinking was causing nearly all my problems for me, my relationships, my work self, and for my family, I began to explore literature, podcasts, sobriety apps. I eventually found the book *We Are the Luckiest* and subsequently "The Luckiest Club" online sobriety support group, and several sub-groups.

I learned that I had landed in a safe place. I could swear, sob, laugh, and be supported. I learned that if I listened, I would hear all the elements of my story as others shared. It was incredibly comforting to learn that I was not alone. No self-deprecating feeling, I had of shame or guilt or doubt was unique to me. The community shared these feelings. I was not alone.

In fact, because my feelings were more or less normal or natural in the community, I was better able to face them. The community gave me permission to feel those feelings and to say them out loud and know that I would be accepted instead of judged.

With our shared experiences, the group reminded me that while my emotions are part of me, I am not the sum of my emotions. While I felt shame and guilt from my past, no one in the group was ashamed of me. This empathy and acceptance changed my life—and probably saved it. The messages that I am not alone, that no one is ashamed of me, that by showing up and sharing my voice I am where I need to be today has sustained me in my journey.

So, without community, there is a good chance I would be divorced, estranged from my children, and possibly out of a job. With community, I have found the support to accept myself, give myself grace, and turn my life around. My wife and I are back in love, my children seek me out for games and activities, and are neither embarrassed by, nor ashamed of, me.

"The work" we all need to do in recovery can be enigmatic. Some communities (TLC) provide unconditional love and compassion and a venue to be heard and supported. Others provide a pathway in the form of steps (AA), and others (Lionrock) literally give written assignments (Phase work) to help guide members on their journey. Not every recovery program is right for everyone, but every program is right for someone. The thing they all share is community—they give opportunity to open your soul to fellow travelers and know you will be met with compassion.

If you want to go fast, travel alone. If you want to go far, travel together.

SARA PINGREE

Oncology nurse, wife, mother, and member of TLC and the Pandemic Sober Squad. Retired people-pleaser who now loves mornings (no hangovers!) and watching the birds.

Before I got sober more than two years ago, my life felt like a rollercoaster. One day I would fly high, feeling confident and strong. Then, the next day I would plummet into despair with no way out. My life felt out of control as it was filled with daily lies to my husband, Andy, and our boys.

I would wear multiple masks a day in an effort to give those around me the version of Sara they expected. Nearly every day, I would go to work with a strong resolve to do things differently, but at the end of the day, I would walk to my car, exhausted from wearing all those masks. Knowing I had a second shift waiting for me at home, filled with kids activities and homework, dinner, and other daily chores, I would head right to the convenience store for a pack of cigarettes and beer.

A pit would form in my stomach with a feeling of, "This isn't who I am," but I was unable to stop myself. I wanted to check out. I wanted to bury my emotions. Arriving home with glossy eyes, perfume sprayed hair, and a long list of excuses for my tardiness, I would attempt this tightrope walk of "Everything is fine, I'm fine" to my husband and two boys.

Andy was adept at spotting my inebriation, which would undoubtedly lead to an evening-long fight with his trying to get me to admit I had been drinking and my flat-out lying. I spent years in denial—in denial to him and myself.

I tried for a long time to find that third door Laura McKowen writes of in her book, *We Are the Luckiest*. I was willing to do anything except quit drinking. Alcohol couldn't possibly be the problem, not *my* problem. I would moderate. I would quit smoking. I would only drink on the weekends. I would only drink beer, no wine. I would only drink socially, not alone. I would leave my money at home.

I made these hollow promises over and over again to my family and myself. Reading Laura's book was the god-shot I needed to finally admit it was truly time—for fucking real this time—to quit drinking.

I have learned a lot about myself since getting sober. The gifts I have received in sobriety are beyond anything I could've ever imagined. I am still the same person at my center, but the way I look at life has completely changed. I no longer run away from my life, no longer chase my fear of missing out, and I care significantly less about others' opinions of me.

I have discovered that at the center of my addiction is people-pleasing. As an Enneagram 2, The Helper, I care deeply about those close to me—or even the neighbor down the road. I want to provide for them at the detriment of my own mental health.

The emotional sobriety work of recovery has given me the tools to recognize my people-pleasing patterns and to change how I interact with others. I am learning for the first time in my life to stand up for myself.

My daily habits and patterns play a big role in this work. The first thing I did to get sober was to join The Luckiest Club. It took me out of my solo, shame-filled space of "I must fix this myself" to enter a world of women and men who felt the same way I did.

Having a community has provided the biggest impact on my

recovery. I have made connections and friendships that will last a lifetime. I attend multiple meetings a week and in talking about the trials and tribulations of sobriety with likeminded friends, I keep sobriety at the center of my daily life.

A commonly heard quote in the recovery community is "The opposite of addiction isn't sobriety, it's community," by Johann Hari. I feel this in my core. Another game changer for me has been writing in a journal each day or "word vomit" as I like to call it since nothing is beautiful about my string of thoughts except that they are out of my brain and on the paper.

Julia Cameron, author of *The Artist's Way,* calls this practice "Morning Pages." I take this very seriously and write daily, sometimes for only a few minutes and other times for an hour, while I sit outside on my porch. It puts me in touch with my heart and soul. Through writing, I dig deep and discover thoughts and feelings I didn't even know needed to come to the surface.

Lastly, time in nature, although not a daily pattern, has given me much joy and gratitude. I take walks that I call my nature baths—where my only goal is to walk slowly and notice every detail big and small surrounding me. I immerse myself in the beauty nature has given us. It provides me with feelings of wonder and awe, and I always return home with comfort and a solid footing of my place in this big, beautiful world.

In many ways, my relationships in sobriety have improved greatly, and in others ways, it continues to be a struggle. I am fortunate enough to have a few close friends who completely understood and accepted me when I told them about my struggles with alcohol.

The relationship with my husband, on the other hand, continues to be filled with ups and downs. When I was drinking heavily, I was consumed with such shame and distrust of myself that I defaulted all choices and decisions to him. I turned our marriage into a parent/child relationship.

Recovering from people-pleasing has been the main work of my emotional sobriety, and unsurprisingly it shows up most in my relationship with Andy. When I speak up for myself in our marriage now, sometimes this frustrates him, and he resists my words as he gets used to a different wife. We both must work hard to learn new ways to effectively communicate. Getting sober has greatly improved our relationship on so many levels but it has also left us with a new unsteadiness that we are still trying to figure out. It continues to be a work in progress.

As I mentioned earlier, when I was drinking, I felt as though I had no control over my emotions and that they would swing wildly from one extreme to the other. Getting sober hasn't magically made all the difficult times disappear, but I am now able to face them with equanimity. I am able to take a deep breath, name my emotions, and recognize that they, too, shall pass.

I have discovered an evenness or a balance to my emotions. I can see them and not have an immediate aversion to them. They no longer overwhelm me, or if they do, I can process the hard emotions without spiraling or getting hooked.

Yung Pueblo, in his book, *Lighter,* says, "Since the amount of stress you experience depends on the intensity of your reaction, the only solution that is within your control is changing yourself."

Learning this new self-awareness has changed my energy from one of survival to one of growth. I can now honestly say that my life is wholehearted, expansive, and full of grace.

This work, the work of recovery and emotional sobriety is hard. It is a slow and difficult reveal to your true being, but please know that it is a thousand percent worth it.

Begin today. What are you waiting for?

ANN P.

Grateful and proud mother of two amazing sons and nana to my incredible grandson and granddaughter. Resilient, grief surviving joy seeker.

As I entered my third year of sobriety and reflected on my journey, if someone would have told me that I would stop drinking, I would have said they were crazy. I was the person who couldn't understand how someone could go to a restaurant without having a glass of wine or another drink.

Was I being judgmental? Of course, I was. How boring their lives must be, and how in the world could they have fun without alcohol? And if they were not drinking, they surely "had a problem" with alcohol or they were a raging alcoholic and must have hit rock bottom, which forced them to quit drinking

I drank occasionally my whole life, though after my first marriage of nearly 29 years ended in 2011, it picked up. I began with a glass or two, but over time one glass became two and before you know it, it turned into a bottle. I didn't consume that much every night, but certainly not just on the weekend. A year after my divorce, I moved across country and remarried in late 2014 after a two-year long-distance relationship, though we didn't live together until August 2015. I thought my life was going so well, but I couldn't have been more wrong.

On December 22, 2015, my life changed forever, and the memory of that day is seared into my memory. On a normal Tuesday evening, my ex-husband called to tell me our youngest son was dead. He was only 30 and died alone in a weekly motel.

I can still feel the guttural scream coming out of my mouth like it was yesterday. *This can't be happening.* But it was and I didn't have to wait for the death certificate to know his death was a result of over a decade of drinking.

The death certificate confirmed it—end stage liver disease due to chronic ethanol abuse. And if you are thinking, *Isn't ethanol what we put in our vehicles?* you are right. When we drink alcohol, it is like drinking gasoline; although I didn't really get it until I quit drinking.

Most people would assume after you lose your child as a result of alcohol abuse, you would stop drinking. I didn't, in fact, after his funeral I drank two bottles of wine. Losing him was the worst thing I had ever experienced. While from the outside it appeared I was okay, I wasn't. The grief of losing him was unbearable and the only way I could cope was to drink. It numbed the pain enough for me to survive each day.

Six months after his death, my oldest son's wife was diagnosed with breast cancer. Again, another reason to stop drinking, yet I didn't. I drank even more, as it helped to numb the pain. And to be honest, I didn't think I had a problem with drinking. Everyone drank a glass or two of wine every night, didn't they?

The journey to my rock bottom began in late December 2019 when a traumatic event occurred in my family. It led to a fracture in my relationship with my oldest son and his family. In February 2020, he told me that I was depressed, unhappy, exhibited passive-aggressive behavior, and I had not been present for him in his childhood. He said I acted the same way with my then-six-year-old grandson. He could not let that be repeated with his children. If I did not get therapy, I could not be a part of his life.

This was devastating. I had already lost one son, and I was at risk of losing another. This loss was worse because I knew my youngest was never coming back, yet he was here and losing him was too much to bear. My grandson, who was not quite two when I lost my son, was the reason I survived his death. He gave me a reason to wake up every day. The thought of never seeing him and my unborn granddaughter ever again was unacceptable. Though I didn't know at the time, this was the beginning of my journey to sobriety.

I knew if I wanted to have a relationship with my son, I would have to get help, so I started therapy in mid-March 2020. COVID–19 hit the following week. My drinking escalated exponentially.

Drinking was the only way I could deal with pain of being estranged from my son and his family. Wine and vodka became my only source of comfort. I knew something had to change when I began hiding bottles of vodka under the frozen vegetables in the freezer and started sneaking swigs of that vodka throughout the weekend days. Day drinking during the workweek was off limits, but I knew if something didn't change, I would break that boundary. It took six months of therapy for me to understand that if I had any hope of a reconciliation, I would have to stop drinking. I had my last drink on October 24, 2020.

My intention was to stop drinking on my own, but the next day, a SoberSis Facebook ad popped up to participate in a 21-day reset from alcohol, and I signed up. I believe it was divine intervention. I followed it with a 10-week course on living an alcohol-free lifestyle that gave me the insight into why I had started drinking in the first place. Through SoberSis, I met a group of amazing women, my Juno sisters, who saw me through my darkest days and have become some of my closest friends. Meeting them in person was an experience I will always cherish.

A little over a year after I quit drinking, I joined TLC (The Luckiest Club), an online sobriety support community. In TLC, I've connected with more women, my Crone sisters, that have become close friends as well. And I've been blessed to meet some of them in real life. Connection was the key to my breakup with alcohol.

Giving up alcohol was the first step, and if I'm being honest, for me, was the easy part. The real work began was becoming emotionally sober. I had to face things I had suppressed for my entire life, which was difficult, and I am still working through them. I had to take a long, and often painful, look at my behavior and how it affected my family and those around me. I faced the fact that everything my son said about me was true. I have an enormous amount of guilt and regret in how I have behaved in the past and am still in therapy working to become a better person. I've learned more in the years since I got sober than I had in the previous 60.

Some might say that their life is over when they hit rock bottom. For me it was just the opposite. The death of one son and near loss of another were the two worst moments of my life and catalyst to my sobriety journey. My son's honesty saved my life, and I am forever grateful that he loved me enough to tell me the truth. If not for him, I am certain I would still be drinking and hurting the people whom I love most in this world. I know I would still be estranged from him had I not gotten sober and been in therapy, as it was an integral part of my recovery.

Sobriety truly gave me a new lease on life, one I see with so much clarity. Sobriety has changed me so much in the last three years. My marriage ended, and I am starting my life all over again. I'm rebuilding my relationship with my son and being a part of his life is the very best part of sobriety. Is it perfect? No, of course not, but it's mine. I'm grateful and blessed for what I have and look forward to what lies ahead.

TAMMI SCOTT

Recent retiree. Seeker and facilitator of healthy, meaningful connection. Practitioner and student of holding space. Yogi, writer, sublime human.

To help you understand what I learned through my alcohol-free communities: Narcotics Anonymous (NA), Alcoholics Anonymous (AA), She Recovers, Served Up Sober, and currently The Luckiest Club (TLC), I first need to tell you a little about who I was—or who I wasn't—when I first got sober.

I had no clue who I really was because I was a compilation of pretty much anyone in my orbit. That included my charming, but absent, verbally and physically abusive, alcoholic father; my emotionally unavailable, stressed-out, verbally, and physically abusive mother; and any and all friends or relatives I desperately wanted to be like because I hated being me. I was a 28-year-old single mother of three lovely young children, and I had failed at every single role I tried to fulfill. I was dangerously close to dying from a lifetime of slow, destructive, spiritual decay. Astoundingly enough, I had no clue that my drug and alcohol use since age 11 was contributing to this demise.

However, when a psychiatrist referred me to a center for

alcohol and addiction, I embraced the recommendation with a deep sense of elated relief. There was a name for what was wrong with me! I complied with all their conditions: attend group therapy, individual sessions with a counselor and, *gulp,* attend 12-step meetings.

Suddenly I recalled another therapist who had gotten me to briefly try antidepressants several years earlier and had handed me a list of AA meeting locations "to try." But I had never given it any credence at the time since I was trying to fix my depression—I don't even think I stayed on the medication for a week. It made me feel too tired and like I was underwater.

What I experienced from NA and AA took me an extremely long time to trust. Unconditional acceptance, attention, listening, love, and a god of my understanding, which at the time felt like good orderly direction in the form of the 12-steps and meeting attendance. My first 12-step meeting was a women's step study in Narcotics Anonymous. The format alternated weeks between open sharing and step study, which gave me a solid foundation for what principles and values they imparted. Before then, I hadn't ever given principles and values any real consideration.

I learned what a powerful paradox surrender can be, and was, for me. I came to know I could be seen, heard, and accepted unconditionally—as I was. I learned that honesty, open minded-ness, and willingness were a trifold foundation for profound personal and spiritual growth and transformation.

I didn't just learn the principles and virtues of honesty, hope, faith, courage, integrity, willingness, humility, brotherly love, discipline, perseverance, spirituality, and service; I started to live them. This helped me become a better parent, friend, family member, employee, human, and recovering alcoholic.

I came to think of 12-step meetings as circles of healing. I was soon able to recognize other circles and communities of healing outside of AA. At the time, I had been sober for 19 years and they were principally yoga and writing circles. While those communities were not alcohol-free, they were an important bridge to myself and to the world at large beyond my 12-step community.

Through the contemplative, embodied practice of yoga and the personal exploration of writing my stories, my truths, and my journey, I began to discover and embrace who I was beyond the good alcoholic/addict that NA and AA helped me become. I'd started to drift away from 12-step meetings because I wasn't finding the sense of belonging and acceptance I used to. I couldn't verbalize it, but I felt it and continued to slowly pull away.

The She Recovers Foundation came on to my social media radar because another woman whose page I followed on Facebook had attended a She Recovers New York convention the previous year. Suddenly I saw a lot more posts about this Canadian mother/daughter duo who founded an organization for women in recovery from anything. Their philosophy and motto is that "everyone is recovering from something," which I believed to be true.

I was drawn to and intrigued by the foundation. I expressed interest in a convention She Recovers was having nearby in Los Angeles in 2018, but I had a few concerns that I voiced respectfully on their post about the lack of women of color as convention speakers. To my surprise, one of the founders, Mama Dawn, contacted me directly to address my concerns!

We set up a time to have tea and to have a deeper discussion over the phone later that day. During our call, she was warm, open, and so supportive. She recommended two women of color in sobriety who were beginning their own communities and events near me in San Diego.

One of the women of color was named Shari Hampton of Served Up Sober. She was a quietly dynamic, queer, sober woman who posted short inspirational Instagram videos and provided meditation and restorative nutrition classes at a community building in San Diego. Other women of color in the community facilitated the classes, and I learned a lot about expanding my own recovery to include whole body wellness practices. A restorative eating coach gave monthly cooking classes using healthy, nutritious foods and called it "love made edible." The meditation classes were weekly, and Shari facilitated a Saturday morning Zoom call for women of color in recovery. I was loved my experiences with Served Up Sober.

Shari was studying to become a She Recovers Recovery Coach and helped me apply for a scholarship to attend the She Recovers 2019 Creating Connections tour. At this event, I got to practice yoga with co-founder, Taryn Strong, and got to meet with Mama Dawn face-to-face.

During her testimony about her recovery journey, Taryn Strong spoke about trying to attend 12-step meetings in her early sobriety, but she never felt as good leaving an AA meeting as she did after a yoga class. So she made yoga a central part of her recovery.

My heart raced with recognition at the truth of her words. I started drifting away from my 12-step meetings because I felt better after yoga classes too! Later I talked with Mama Dawn about this revelation that made me feel guilty and disloyal to my 12-step community. She explained that she has found sobriety and recovery outside of NA and AA, so she doesn't always go to their meetings either.

What I learned from Taryn and Mama Dawn's experiences that day helped me understand my own liberation and possibilities for my sobriety independent of AA, where I didn't fit anymore— even though I owed a world of debt to AA for teaching me so much about principles and values, for giving me a design for living for a while.

Four months later, the COVID–19 pandemic shut down the world in March 2020. In response to this frightening, uncertain, and chaotic time, I seemed to shut down as well. My home yoga studio shut down. I couldn't bring myself to do any yoga at home by myself, and I didn't want to do it online.

I was shaken enough to try attending some of the online 12-step meetings, but I still didn't feel connected. I felt untethered and so alone. And while I didn't want any alcohol or mind-altering substances, I was in deep trouble emotionally and maybe even mentally.

Then a friend reached out and invited me to share my story for a recovery meeting she facilitated. Her friend, Laura McKowen, author of *We Are The Luckiest,* had been hosting online sobriety support meetings since we'd all been cooped up. I said yes because it was my friend, and AA taught me to never turn down an opportunity to be of service when asked.

She described what the meetings were like, but I wasn't paying close attention. I'd said yes, I knew how to tell my story. On Friday May 22, 2020, I showed up in a Zoom room of more than 200 people to tell my story. I loved the format of the meeting. I told my story, and after 20-plus years in recovery, I knew how to tell it.

There was a mutual love fest between the TLC community and me that day. I signed up right after the meeting. My friend messaged Laura, and I was hired to be a community moderator for their online forum. My friend received messages from the community asking for me to come back to tell more of my story—Demanding Tammi 2.0.

In the meantime, I'd exchanged emails with the founder, Laura McKowen, and I was attending these amazing recovery meetings where there was no dogma—we showed up as who we were with no labels. Within eight days, Laura hired me to facilitate TLC meetings. And I found what I didn't know was missing: *community*. TLC was like living water for my soul.

MARK HOWER

Traveler. Art museums. New York City. Golf. Tennis. Father of two wonderful women. The long-term illness of my late wife was my excuse.

I must remember that I am an alcoholic. This is my number one priority every day. No question.

I have a relative who has been sober for over 50 years, and this is one of his simple pieces of advice: If I don't take the first drink, I don't get drunk.

I have to remember it *every* day. Even after eight years in recovery. I can be "in recovery" but I can't forget why I am there. I have a daily reminder every morning in the form of an email I receive at 4 a.m. each day. I was invited to join this email list early in my recovery when I attended an AA meeting in Northern Virginia. It often has a "meme" with a recovery-oriented message along with references to AA literature—readings for the day. Also, the email lists congratulations to members of that meeting who are having annual sober anniversaries that day.

I can't say I read the materials that often anymore, but here's the point: I generally at least glance at my email on my phone before I get out of bed, so even if I don't read that email, I am reminded that I am receiving that email, and continue to receive it for a reason: I am an alcoholic and before my feet hit the floor, I get that reminder that nothing can be improved that day by having a drink.

If I complained about the time spent going to meetings, my first AA sponsor would point out that I spent hours and hours and hours each day drinking—is it that difficult to spend *one hour* at a meeting? He also suggested getting to half a meeting was better than no meeting. You might hear one thing you needed to hear or say one thing that someone else needed to hear in that thirty minutes.

Memories I might want to forget. I have to remember the worst days that led me to start my recovery journey. I never want to be there again. People often talk about the lows—the bottom they reached—that led them to give up alcohol and start living another way. My lows were mental more than anything and I don't *ever* to go there again.

Connection and participation. I have to be connected to a community of people who are also living without alcohol—those who *don't* pick up a drink every day. It took me a long time to realize how important this is. I did not want to share my story or any thoughts about how I felt. That stunted my growth and took my recovery longer to get started. Once I learned to share and learn from others, the magic started to happen.

Every day I think about what meetings are available and what meetings to attend. If I don't think I will get to a live meeting, I will get to an online meeting. *Meeting makers make it.*

Pick up the phone. I recently moved to the woods after spending my whole life in urban or suburban areas. Finding human interaction there is harder. I can go to online meetings, but nothing is better than picking up the phone and speaking with someone. Text works, too, but doesn't quite do it for me. Talking to someone about the thoughts ruminating in my mind is the best place for me to move on.

Speaking. I speak in two ways. One is to briefly share my thoughts at a meeting or "lead" a meeting by telling my story for twenty or thirty minutes. The goal is to share my experience, strength, and hope. While I will often talk about the progression of my drinking and its negative impacts on my life, I feel it is more important to share my recovery journey, its trials and tribulations, and when things get better.

Sometimes getting better takes a while. Someone who drank as long as I did may need quite some time for a mental and physical transition. It can be like learning to breathe again. I talk about things that help me stay sober. Finally, I hope to show how good my life is in sobriety to help others see that sobriety is worthwhile. I believe that if a person can't find joy and happiness, he or she will look to the drink again. I hope my life will show that people can achieve sobriety .

Sometimes after I speak someone will say, "Thank you for sharing your story, Mark. It was what I needed tonight," or "What you said in the meeting will keep me sober today."

These comments keep *me* sober.

Merry bands of meeting makers. I often visit meetings while I'm traveling. I'm not the "Johnny Appleseed" of AA or recovery in general, but I enjoy seeing how different meetings are run and hearing new voices. It is great to be welcomed into a group because we are all in this together. I've been told a great message I carry is that I am comfortable enough in myself to walk into other meetings—I have no fear and expect to be welcomed as a fellow traveler. Also, going to meetings is important enough to me that I search them out when I travel. I also offer the gift of a fresh voice in the room.

Social media. I do not trumpet my sober life on social media, but I am connected to a lot of people whom I have encountered on my sober journey. To see that they are doing well makes me happy.

Boundaries. In one recovery group I was in, at each meeting we set a goal for that day. Inevitably, one member said he would "stay in his own lane." It took me a while to understand the importance of this. For years, I was extremely empathetic. I was good at listening, but I internalized everyone else's problems, which added to my own anxiety and depression.

This especially happened when I was the caregiver for my late wife during her illness. In the first year of my first go at sobriety, I had been the caretaker for my parents and fell into anxiety and depression. That was one of the reasons why I had a major relapse after fourteen months of sobriety. In my second round of sobriety, which has been continuous, I did again help care for my parents, but I put some space between them and me. A couple of family members pointed out that my keeping my distance would benefit all of us in the end. I could enjoy my final years with my parents without it again bringing me down. My boundaries were a gift in many ways.

Gratitude. When I was mentally crashing before my first attempt at sobriety, I could not make a list of *anything* for which I felt gratitude. I must have gratitude for my sober world. If I don't have joy and happiness, I will drink again. I will spiral down, lose my "emotional sobriety," and pick up a drink. Drinking was my solution to stress for decades, and I know that it would try to become my solution again—if I would let it.

I have to remember that if I am happy today, it is because alcohol is no longer in my life. I don't wake up with a raging hangover. I don't lose days because I feel so terrible. I don't make myself "feel better" by picking up a drink and starting the cycle all over. I don't wake up at night and have more drinks to go back to sleep. I don't have to go to the liquor store multiple times a week. I don't have to pay attention to my drinking in case I might have to drive. I don't drink and drive which I did so many times. I don't have to do *any* of this anymore.

Variety. My sobriety journey has had many phases. Perhaps I need variety. Variety of meetings. Variety of readings. Variety of people. The only constant is that I know I can't pick up a drink today. Picking up a drink will improve *nothing*. I enjoy being able to sense a world without vodka or scotch.

New roads. Lately, I have moved outside the traditional world of recovery meetings and community to find different ways to help others. I have joined the board of a recovery non-profit near my home to support its programs to educate and assist individuals, schools, and businesses on substance-abuse disorders. I have also just completed training to be a recovery coach. Not all people respond to the typical avenues for recovery. I hope to help those who need an additional hand.

Every day is not perfect. My world is not perfect. I often remember the words of a psychologist I saw for about a year: **Every day that you are sober is a gift**. Every single one of them. I remember *that* every day.

JANELL KATHRYN SKLAPSKY

A strong and self-assured woman, she carries the wisdom of knowing herself. Her journey has led her through challenging and transformative experiences, where grief has been a profound teacher, unveiling the extraordinary beauty that coexists with pain. Immersed in somatic work for the past seven years, she continues to deepen her studies under the guidance of a mentor. With deep trust in her own healing journey and a connection to the red road and ceremony way of life, she supports her fellow travelers towards trust in themselves, life. and their own becoming.

I am proud that I have become a woman who follows the call of her spirit, a woman who listens to, and is learning to believe in, her prayer.

My becoming sober began by my being brave enough to see the prayer that was hidden in my heart—to be sober and to live a different way. Alcohol and substances kept me swimming in pain rather than letting it be a teacher and catalyst for transformation, beauty, and becoming.

When that prayer in my heart was revealed to me, I was shaky and oh-so-tender. When I chose to follow it I was scared and sure.

I knew there was a path before me, and all I had to do was stay on it.

My journey has not been perfect, but I have learned it was never supposed to be. Perfection was a heavy armor that I wore. With space and loving presence, I have set that heaviness down and come to give myself and my system the chance to rest well in the imperfection and messiness of life as it is and myself as I am.

"In this moment, all is okay," are words that I held onto for a time as I felt my way forward. And when things weren't okay, and there were certainly times like that, and there still are, I learned I could, and I can ask for help. Each time I have put that call out, the help has come—whether from a friend, family, stranger, my own inner uprightness and strength, or through the mysterious workings of a prayer answered.

I once heard a Lakota elder say that when you make a prayer to remember it, so that when the answer makes its way to you, you can recognize it. Another teacher shared to not put doubt on my prayer. To set that down and to believe because it wouldn't work otherwise.

Some of the hardest and most remarkable lessons have been when the answers to those prayers I most wanted answered did not come in the way I would have hoped. Oh, how that has ached at times. And oh, how that has taught me—and is teaching me, to let go.

When I force, control, or hold on tight, I get far away from myself and the way that is mysteriously mine and meant for me.

When I let go, I am held, and I can lean back into life's gracious holding.

I have seen signs of that holding along the way—heart rocks found along the path, songs on the radio in the grocery store or gas station; those seemingly small signs that I am right where I am meant to be.

And then in grand and magic moments my spirit has called me forward in undeniable and unexpected ways. To look away in these moments would mean to shut down and turn away from myself and from God's speaking directly to and through me.

That's how it was when I first got the call to Sun Dance in 2019. I had been starting to learn an Indigenous ceremony way of life after feeling a pull to it since I was young. I would attend the ceremony, help, and support—but I never envisioned participating in the Sun Dance myself. Yet, when the call came it was so clear in my being that I took the next step. A subtle part of me knew that this would change everything. Little did I know that there would be change that would hurt. That would be hard. And that would open my eyes, heart, mind, and spirit to a beauty beyond words, shape or form.

I am proud of my willingness to listen to that kind of call. To go towards what may not be easy but is nonetheless meant for me.

In my early 20s, that seed was already awakening. I got my first of many tattoos, marking my wrist with the ancient Latin words, *Nosce Te Ipsum*, meaning, "To know thyself."

Those words came at a time when I truly did not know myself. And yet, when I heard them, my spirit clearly spoke: "Go this way."

And as I have gone this way—mine—and learned to trust my own unique path, my listening has refined and grown through each step and each falter. A desire to keep my light strong in a world that has much ugliness has taken form. A desire to continue to believe in and feel into the beauty and good that is still ever present and real. The prayer that is alive in me now, the call that is softly making itself known, is that I might continue along the path of dropping into belief—a belief so strong in that good— not for myself, but for those who stand at a distance from it, from themselves and the prayer hidden in their own hearts. May somehow, some way that be revealed to them, and may there be enough of a spark of belief and light along the path that they, too, might be brave enough to experience, know and trust in the possibility and holding of life—and that voice that is ready and waiting to tell them to "go this way," the way that is mysteriously theirs and meant for them. May these words and this prayer go where it needs to go. Love, Dharamjeev.

JENNIFER BRIDGMAN

Woman. Wife. Sober Warrior. Three-boy mama. Three-cat mama. Writer. Student of life and myself. Enneagram 2. Nature lover. Music lover. Horse lover. Philanthropist. Peer support mentor for families new to paralysis/spinal cord injury. Saying "no" to alcohol to "yes" to life since August 2020.

A Leading Lady
By Jennifer Bridgman

It's hard to say when exactly I'd lost the starring role in my own life story—when alcohol took center stage, and I became the unwitting understudy.

Looking back, I cannot pinpoint any pivotal event or dramatic plot twist when everything seemed to change.

What I can assure you is that I loved booze right from the start, and for many years, I believed it loved me back. But I lost my starring role over time, not overnight. A few years perhaps. It's hard to say, considering the slippery, indistinct trajectory. Addiction is tricky like that.

As with many people, my drinking began as a joyous and

connective thing. In my teens, I became known as a girl who could drink and that became a key part of my identity. Something I celebrated and a source of pride. But as the years progressed, drinking became something that I desired and depended upon too much—often to a destructive degree. Over time, I became known as a girl who couldn't drink. And that, too, became part of my identity—one loaded with shame. To be someone who can't "drink responsibly" in an alcohol-loving society is a tough spot to be in. Rather than turn on booze, I turned on myself. "Sober" was the ugliest word I knew. I was devastated and humiliated that this had become my thing. Over the next decade, I oscillated between periods of drinking and abstinence—secretly loathing myself throughout both. While alcohol caused undeniable confusion, pain, and strain on my relationships, not drinking also hurt. It left me feeling like a flawed, sad outcast, the color beige in a technicolor world. Throughout both my years of active addiction and my years of white-knuckle sobriety, it's no wonder I suffered in silence; I was on the losing team either way.

Ultimately, it took 10 years of stumbling through the miserable moderation routine for me to get it—"it" being my wholly wanting and celebrating sobriety. Putting down the drink was one thing—and a brutal one at that—but genuine healing and transformation were only possible once I began to own my story in a way that it no longer owned me. The (condensed) story I am about to share contains tough truths I'd planned on taking to the grave—and nearly did. But instead of an early death, I survived addiction and learned how to thrive in recovery. I am wildly proud to have reclaimed the starring role in my own life story. And I'm here to promise you that you can, too.

Act One: Setting the Stage

I began drinking in my teens—the summer before my sophomore year, to be exact. I was a naïve, 14-year-old, braces-wearing dreamer who had never tasted alcohol, driven a car, or had a serious boyfriend. Within a year, all of that would change. For me, booze was an undeniable love at first sip—although it's safe to say that I never quite "sipped" anything again after that first keg party. In my small, insulated bubble of a hometown in Northern California, "partying" was not only accepted but also respected. A few of my girlfriends were already experimenting with alcohol, so in a sense I felt figuratively late to the party. Back then, it seemed your whole life could change by missing or attending a single rager. I felt an incessant need to claim my seat at the table and make up for lost time.

I was in high school during the mid-90s. A time of Pearl Jam and Dr. Dre. Of keg parties and flannel shirts and red Solo Cups. Of mix tapes and passed notes in class. We threw house parties, ran from police through the woods, attended Grateful Dead shows whenever they rolled into town, and basically did dangerous, foolish things with few consequences. I continued to get good-enough grades and play varsity sports. I had a loving family, good friends, and the boyfriend. But even then, I knew I drank differently. One day you'll have to deal with this, I whispered to myself in rare moments of honest reflection. But that hypothetical one day never became today.

Ironically, my drinking did initially lend me tremendous power. It allowed me to feel at ease within my own skin—something I secretly did not feel, despite trying to appear otherwise. I longed to love and to be loved in return without a clue how to go about it. I desperately wanted to be included and appreciated. To be known and to matter in the world—and booze seemed to be the surefire shortcut to all these things.

By my twenties, I subconsciously prioritized and protected my drinking at all costs. After college, I moved to Hollywood with my Rock 'n' Roll musician boyfriend, hours away from my family, which made it easier to conceal my addiction. I surrounded myself with people who drank like me—or at least wouldn't look too closely at my habits. For several years, I held a solid marketing position with a television network, but I was increasingly wrapped up by the bright lights and dizzying nights of the Sunset Strip. I'd suffer through brutal hangovers at the office, praying the eye drops, Tylenol, and Listerine would co-sign my secrets as I pretended my unraveling world was all stitched up. It was easy to minimize and trivialize booze-related consequences in my environment. I hid my alcohol addiction from the world as best I could—which was shockingly well. Very few people, including those I loved or even lived with, knew the real amount of time I spent drinking, thinking about drinking, thinking about not drinking, or recovering from drinking.

I had become a shell of a person, trapped in an unhealthy relationship which only further reinforced my understudy role. Booze both brought us together and tore us apart. I stayed because I drank, and I drank because I stayed—until things grew irreparable and abusive, as tends to happen in alcohol-soaked unions. And when my ex finally moved out, and I found myself living alone for the first time in my life, booze moved in like never before.

Act Two: Masks and Moderation

By the age of 29, I'd fallen in love with a beautiful man worthy of my future and whole heart. Despite my fears of being seen—flaws and all—I began to lower my walls. It didn't take long for him to see me clearly: a woman he loved, trapped in serious addiction. Eventually there was an intervention and an ultimatum and a trip to rehab. I did manage to quit drinking, but I never managed to quit the secrets, including the biggest one of all: I never actually wanted sobriety—I just didn't want to lose the guy. I continued to ache for alcohol, haunted by its memory everywhere I looked. My husband and I proceeded to build a beautiful life together, a golden-hued one beyond my wildest dreams, complete with three wondrous children. And yet, I remained secretly heartbroken backstage. I told no one this. I couldn't—not with all the blessings in my life and the hell I'd already put others through. I didn't believe anyone could understand me. After all, I couldn't understand me. What kind of deranged fool continued to covet something that had left such a wake of destruction? I couldn't figure out how to abandon the drink, so I learned to abandon myself further.

Alcohol returned, steadily and scarily. It remained my greatest reward at the end of any given day, long after the drinking stopped being rewarding. I chose alcohol night after night, until it was no longer a choice I had to make.

I survived in this unsustainable space for several years. I was convincing—talented even—as I settled for being the understudy. But just beneath the curated surface, my heart ached for bigger dreams left unanswered. I acted out most scenes with my insides not matching my outsides, knowing that I was never truly connecting with others because I relied heavily on masks and props. As much as I longed for my moment in the spotlight, I was terrified of being fully seen. I felt like a fraud playing my own part. Because I was.

Act Three: Reclaiming the Light

Today, I consider myself part of a modern-day revolution in which we understand that becoming addicted to an addictive substance is just one of many things that can happen to a perfectly imperfect human. We aim to not only shed light on the true nature of addiction, but also on what genuine recovery looks like as well. While each of us has a unique journey, we don't have to travel alone. We are not inherently flawed, nor are we forever defined by the worst things we've done. Most of us in recovery consider ourselves the luckiest people we know, for once you've experienced true darkness and reclaimed the light, the view will never look the same.

There are many reasons females like me learn to shrink on life's stage. Often our concurrent roles of woman, wife, mother, and helper-to-all feel at odds with our leading lady status, as we are bombarded with reminders that our primary duties fall under the supporting role category. I was supposed to be the fixer with the answers, not the one with the problem and questions. My female roles indeed kept me suffering in silence, afraid to blow the whistle on myself and ask for help. But the single most disempowering thing I ever did was put alcohol to my own lips.

One day, when I least expected it, I found my Day One. Or

rather it found me: my own body staged an intervention. Some may call it pancreatitis; I prefer to call it the gift of crisis. I became unwilling to live another moment in the agony of addiction, and my walls came crashing down. So how did I do it? The only way. The hard way—right through it. I left my dark, isolated seat back-stage and began to take up space on the stage. I studied and rehearsed and flubbed countless lines, but I kept showing up for myself. I continued to whisper "yes" to my future self as my inner fear continued to scream "no." Months added up. I began to redis-cover joy, connection, and genuine pride in myself. I stopped looking over my shoulder in regret and looked ahead into the unknown with a gleam in my eye. I quit straining my eyes to find approval from the audience and began to look inward.

I surrendered to the reality that life has no dress rehearsal, and as a result, I became forever unwilling to settle for smaller roles that no longer served me. Today, I am learning to stare back into the spotlight in all my unique glory, unflinching and unafraid to shine. I'm learning it's safe to reveal my quirks and questions, my wrinkles and wounds, and all my beautiful scars. I understand that even when life hands me a challenging script, I still retain personal freedom and agency to make it my own. I have become fluent in the language of truth and vulnerability, keenly aware that my pauses are just as potent as my prose.

As a leading lady, I have learned that it's important to know my lines but even better to know my character. I know that my story is still being written, and it will have many acts; some will be full of love, others full of lessons. I am aware that I must savor the light but not shun the dark—as both are requirements for being human. Each day I make a choice to remain dignified and true in mind, body, and spirit.

It required getting sober to see the sobering truth: that for decades I'd been the understudy—not the star—of my own life story. I'd handed over the script to booze and fear, opting for a backstage seat in the hopes of avoiding pain and gaining love, acceptance, and validation outside of myself. Sometimes it looked like running when I should have stayed. Sometimes it looked like staying when I should have run. But I see now that all my pain served a purpose. That all those wrong turns and dead ends were simply a necessary part of my journey.

Stepping into the light after being my own understudy for so long is a glorious thing. I have peace in my soul that I didn't have before. It comes from a deep knowing that when the curtain closes on my final act, and I find myself standing alone on the stage, I will meet myself with love. For my life story became the greatest one I would ever know—because it was all mine.

KARYN WOMACK

Mom, stepmom, dog mom, wife. Learning and development professional and creative soul. I am happiest when I am next to a body of water and thrive during the summer months. As an Enneagram 2, it took me until my 50s to prioritize taking care of myself (mind, body, soul, and sobriety), and I have never been happier.

Through my recovery, I have consistently seen a therapist. I started seeing her about a year and a half before I stopped drinking, and it was the catalyst to seeing and accepting that alcohol is my thing and there is no healthy way to have it in my life.

In my first year and a half of sobriety I did not have community and did not commit to stopping "forever." I found Brené Brown's TED Talks on sobriety and listened to them every day. I read each of her books in chronological order. I discovered podcasts and listened to Jay Shetty, Lewis Howes, Chase Jarvis, and then Brené Brown, Laura McKowen, and Glennon Doyle. I started following sober people on Instagram, including Holly Whitaker and Laura McKowen, which lead to many others. I bought their books and read every day. I started going to the gym and walking regularly. I started doing transcendental meditation every day.

I had close friends whom I could talk to and be totally honest with, but joining the TLC sober community catapulted my recovery to a different level. It was the first time I realized I was not alone and heard other people put into words what I felt. In three years, I have only gone a handful of days without a virtual meeting. In the heart of the pandemic, I attended multiple meetings a day and still do when I need more connection.

I go through phases of wanting to raise my hand and share during sobriety meetings. Saying words out loud that describe what I'm going through helps me find clarity. I have shared my sobriety story three times, and it has been different each time. The story didn't change, but the way I process the events in my past and my perspective continuously change.

I became the group leader for my state, but another year and a half passed after my joining TLC before I was ready to build friendships and create opportunities to meet people "in real life." It was yet again another level of connection. Some of these friends and I go on trips together, attend sober events, go for walks, meet for coffee, or have a virtual call. It is a genuine friendship on a much deeper level because it isn't about small talk or gossiping.

Change has also been consistent throughout my recovery. There is a saying to "Throw the book at it," which means try everything that might work. I have consistently tried new things. I took two Enneagram courses, the first through my sobriety group. I am an Enneagram 2 which is "The Helper." I didn't believe that for a while, but now it is so obvious. Before sobriety my identity focused on what I could do for other people. It never dawned on me that taking care of myself was the best thing I could do for everyone in my life, especially for me.

Last year I read *The Artist's Way* by Julia Cameron, which is a twelve-week process of exploring our own creativity. One of the practices is taking yourself on an "artist date," which can be anything that helps us unlock our creative process. For me, that looks like going to museums. It inspires me to paint again.

I was a fine arts major in college, and my favorite artist is Vincent Van Gogh. I bought paint and canvases and started painting. I have not painted regularly, but the materials are waiting for me. Another practice is "morning pages," which is three pages of writing whatever comes to mind. The practice allows me to do dump all of my thoughts out on paper. I have always enjoyed writing, and this helps to clear my head.

I read the book *Atomic Habits* by James Clear. The book centers around building good habits and breaking bad ones. His quote, "We don't rise to the level of our goals; we fall to the level of our systems," resonated so much with my recovery. The systems he talks about are daily habits and the power of getting one percent better every day.

I also got his habits journal. There are three parts. The daily prompt is a question of my own choosing every month, such as, "What did I learn today?" The habit tracker is a checklist of daily habits for each month, and the journal is an open section with several ideas for decision-making. This helps me be intentional about my day and what I do. Alcohol is not the only way to escape. I can easily get lost in social media and TV if I am not intentional and aware of what I am doing.

I have a "miracle membership" with self-help author Gabby Bernstein's community and have taken her manifest challenge every January. I would have never considered the concept of manifesting before sobriety, but this practice has helped me to start the year positively way and to open myself to my deepest desires while trusting that the universe is on my side.

The membership also has a weekly coaching exercise, which includes a lesson, affirmation, meditation, and weekend wind down. This helps me to continue to discover myself and how I am changing. My third year of recovery was difficult because what I needed had changed, and I was judging myself for not doing the same things I did in my first year and through the pandemic, when I first discovered community. Having a regular practice helps me to question the stories that I tell myself about my own worthiness.

Recently I discovered astrology and my natal chart. My birthday is in August, and I have identified as a Leo but did not know there is a sun, moon, and rising sign. I am a Leo sun and moon, and my rising sign is Cancer. The moon has always been a powerful force in my life, so it was reassuring to see that in my chart. I also learned the position of the stars and planets when I was born. I have an app on my phone that I check daily. I have also started to pull tarot cards regularly.

I grew up going to a Lutheran church, and my father was a theology major in college. I could always talk to him about my faith, or rather questioning my faith, which I have done for as long as I can remember. Faith has never been easy for me, but I believe there is a "God" or energy beyond my capacity for understanding. I am still discovering what that is and learning to trust my higher power.

This feels like a lot as I'm writing it down, but I can summarize with the most important things or deal breakers for me in sobriety as of right now: Meditate, go to sobriety meetings, connect with sober people, write, read, create, listen to music, move my body, be aware of the food I am eating, spend time alone, and keep learning.

MAUREEN ANDERSON

Maureen Anderson is a wife, mother of four, and serial racquet sports enthusiast. After many years of sober curiosity and making, and breaking, rules around her drinking, she finally quit on August 1, 2020. Maureen is a recovery coach professional and a gray-area drinking coach. She works with women who are questioning their drinking and don't know what to do about it. Her goal is to help smash the stigma around gray-area drinking and reach suffering women so they know they're not alone.

Getting and staying sober has been the work of my life. It requires daily effort, and I'm happy to make that effort.

It wasn't always this way. In the beginning, I held on for dear life, trying to make it to the safety and escape of sleep at the end of each day. I spent a lot of time either questioning my decision to quit drinking or crying. I also listened to sober podcasts, read quit lit, and attended The Luckiest Club meetings, trying to learn the secret formula to quit drinking. The rest of my time was spent figuring out how to function in my "normal life" without the one thing I used for relief.

As far as a "secret formula" for quitting drinking, I eventually learned there is no such thing. I did learn, though, that sobriety is a practice built on a foundation of knowing your core values and doing your best to live in alignment with them. Actually, *that's* the secret formula: knowing your values and doing your best to live by them with integrity.

I think that got me into trouble in the first place—forgetting who I was and what my values were. I moved through life with my head down, doing each next thing I was "supposed to do." I never stopped and, as my good friend Becky Vollmer taught me to ask myself, "How do you feel?" and "What do you need?" I was living out of alignment and using alcohol to numb the pain from being so misaligned. One day, I couldn't take it anymore. I was too tired of hangovers, depression, compulsion, and feeling alone. I had had enough.

So. Since that day I have done the following things to stay sober.

Connect with others who get it. This has been the most effective practice of sobriety. Laura McKowen said, "One stranger who understands your experience exactly will do for you what hundreds of close friends and family who don't understand cannot. It is the necessary palliative for the pain or stretching into change. It is the cool glass of water in hell."

Talking and listening to people who move through this world without using alcohol to cope or celebrate is a balm for what initially feels like a deep wound. To speak your real truth to another person and be met with empathy and understanding calms the nervous system like nothing else can.

Read books that inspire. Since I quit drinking, I've curated a library of books that teach me a new way to live. It began with sober memoirs and has moved to any book that guides me to live with more peace and less tension. Reading wisdom daily keeps my mind forward-thinking and inspired. My collection includes books on positive habits, daily meditation, dopamine, the vagus nerve, poetry, memoirs, neuroscience, the conscious and unconscious mind—you name it, I've got it. Reading five to ten minutes of inspiring words in the morning can set the tone for the day.

Sitting in stillness. I'm committed to carving out a small amount of time each day to unplug, be alone, and focus on nothing but my breath. The practice of releasing my thoughts and coming back to stillness again and again is carrying over into my "real life" and, very slowly, making me less reactive in stressful situations. By sitting in stillness each day I'm developing a spiritual practice and a new way to connect to myself and others. By learning to be calm and comfortable with myself, I can avoid seeking comfort in a glass of wine.

Sleep. This is a big one—especially in the beginning. For at least the first few months of sobriety, I slept 10 hours a night. I couldn't get enough—maybe my body was compensating for all the lost sleep, or maybe the mental exertion of fighting the chronic urge to drink exhausted me. Things have leveled out, and I don't require as much sleep anymore, but it continues to be a priority. When I don't get enough sleep, I have what feels like "brain dehydration." I'm cranky, have less patience, and can't focus. It reminds me of a hangover, and I don't want to live like that anymore. Getting enough sleep is non-negotiable for the quality of life I want to live.

Getting used to being uncomfortable. When I first got sober I did as much as possible to make sure I was comfortable. I bought all my favorite foods, gave myself spa treatments, drank fancy herbal teas, ate the ice cream—treated myself.

I've since learned there's growth in challenging yourself and doing what's uncomfortable. Getting to the other side of an uncomfortable experience builds confidence, resilience, and calmness I've never experienced before.

Socrates said, "The unexamined life is not worth living." Sobriety has compelled me to examine my life, to look under the hood and see what I'm made of. Through self-examination, I've uncovered things I love about myself and things I need to work on.

On a regular basis, I look at the unexpected bonus of getting sober. The hunt for what lights me up; the thrill of finding it. And the sweet release of letting go of what doesn't serve me.

Challenges. Setbacks. Perseverance. Discovery. Knowledge. Success. Growth. These are the rewards of the daily practices I've built into my sober life. What started as making a choice and hoping to not feel terrible anymore turned into a life filled with daily practices that continue to uncover a truer, better way to live.

www.maureenjanderson.com
hello@maureenjanderson.com

MICHAEL WILSON

Joy finder. Purpose seeker. Personal growth coach. Doodle dad and gay hubby. You'll find me at pop diva concerts or musical theater. Once the life of the party, now I simply enjoy life—and chocolate chip cookies.

I am proud I chose me.

I am proud I decided to heal.

I am proud that my goodness before my addiction built a support system around me that wanted to see me succeed.

I am proud I made a decision.

I am proud I pointed myself in the direction of sobriety and of knowing myself more deeply.

I am proud I have done the work—and continue to do the work and will always do the work—to know myself, to heal myself, and to evolve.

I am proud of my vulnerability and lack of fear, of letting people get to know the real Michael.

I am proud of the fact that getting sober wasn't and isn't enough for me.

Getting sober was simply the beginning.

Of what?

Of feeling …

… and understanding my feelings …

… and processing those feelings.

Of getting clear on what my personal values are …

… and understanding how I want to embody my values …

… and how I can design a joyful life around those values.

Of understanding what energized me … and what did not.

Because once I began to understand my feelings, my values, and what energized me, I could begin to know myself. And once I began to know myself, I could get out of my head and into my heart. From there, I could begin to be more present with others.

Presence has been one of the greatest gifts of sobriety. Because I'm more present …

I feel calm.

I feel balanced.

I can focus more acutely.

I procrastinate less.

I empathize with more compassion.

I experience more joy.

I love more deeply.

With more empathy, compassion, and love, I am more patient in difficult situations. And for that, I am truly proud. I am proud that I can more easily regulate myself when things get tough. Because sh*t still gets tough. What I now understand deeply is that it's not about changing what's happening around you, but rather how you respond to what's happening around you.

I am proud of that awareness … of being able to pause when something happens and creating space between it and my response. This allows me to connect with the thoughts and feelings that arise, so I can respond in a way that serves me and supports others.

I am proud of the practices I have adopted that promote my healing, my learning, and my joy. I am proud of…

… my commitment to my yoga practice, which heals body and soul …

... my newly adopted morning meditation, which allows me to practice mindfulness and start the day on my terms ...

... the playtime with my pup, Penny, I have incorporated into my day, which reminds me to reconnect with my inner child that didn't care what others thought of me and had fun ...

... the morning routine with my husband, Brandon, and Penny, where we walk Brandon to work and then head to Dolores Park where Penny runs around with other pups and their humans...

... my investment in myself by attending retreats, workshops, and classes focused on wellness, mindfulness, and self-betterment.

I am proud that in identifying what type of work energizes me, and what doesn't, I have found coaching and facilitation that appreciates my gifts and enables me to help others raise their consciousness so that they can live a more joy-filled and purposeful life. In doing so, I find my life filled with an abundance of joy and purpose. I am proud of the community of joy finders and purpose seekers we are building with the creation of Joyful Gravity.

I am proud that I have given myself permission to live and work authentically, without the need for others' validation.

I am proud that I am now beginning to live the life I always wanted but didn't know I could achieve—or think I deserved.

I can. And I do.

I am proud that I now understand the difference between doing and being. Instead of being what I do, I now do what I am, no longer identifying with what I do, but rather who I am. I am a joy finder. I am a purpose seeker. I am a connector. Understanding this and feeling this has allowed me to operate from a place of love and possibility versus fear. For that I am truly proud, and grateful.

I am proud that I began this journey of sobriety. Of rediscovering myself. Of knowing myself. And of loving myself.

Because once I began to love myself, I could stop looking externally for answers, for validation, or for belonging. I began to trust my instincts and listen to my inner voice, which knows me better than anyone else. That voice, which used to tell me I was different and didn't belong, or that I wasn't good enough or smart enough, was now telling me ...

... I am enough ...

... I have value ...

... I belong ...

... I belong to myself and therefore belong anywhere I am.

I am proud to know me. And proud of who I have grown into. And I'm proud to say that who I am now is the same person I have always been.

Carefree.

Joyful.

Compassionate.

I am proud of the pain I have lived through—and even more proud that I have learned from it. That I have let it inform me and shape me. But not change me.

As a gay man, the word pride invokes a range of emotions. As a young adult, I remember wishing so badly that I wasn't different. Wishing that I weren't gay. Wishing that I could take a pill to make me "normal" or straight. It took me many years to get to a place where I felt truly proud to be gay. Proud to be different. And I thought, at the time, proud to be me. I recall telling my parents years later, that if there were a pill that made me straight, I wouldn't take it after all.

What I didn't realize then was that I faced years of undoing to become truly proud of who I was. And as those emotions arose, I chose not to feel them, and instead I numbed them. It would take almost 20 more years for me to realize that and choose to feel. I'm proud that I made that choice on May 24, 2021.

I stand here now, two years later, proud of so many things.

Proud of decisions I have made.

Proud of practices I have adopted.

Proud of the work I have done.

But most importantly, I stand here proud to be me.

MIKE BREEN

Golf and daily living. Father of two, grandfather of six. Brother, sponsor, mentor. Retired. Formerly in sales, sales management, consulting. Former "All night long"/life of the party/sometimes post party. Other times post party sentimental, sad, fool. Reliable, kind, humorous, honest, trustworthy. Experienced early death of parents—both gone by my age of 18. Lover of sports (football and golf #1) and good jokes. I never say no to a fun meal or coffee with friends or being with grandchildren.

I was full of false pride before I found recovery. I longed for acceptance, adulation, respect, approval, recognition, and appreciation. And I did things to get what I *thought* was all that. I manipulated people to tell me one or more of those things, and alcohol made it easier to compromise the truth, which was that, deep inside, I was a terrified little boy.

My Irish heritage had taught me to "look good at all costs," and I practiced it quite well. Once, without my wife's input, I impulsively put money down on one of the most beautiful homes in our suburb. It featured a circle driveway, oak beam ceilings, and 300 feet of backyard, with a beautiful Japanese Garden. It had all the trappings. People would comment, "Oh, you guys bought that house on Belmont; that is so lovely." I ate all that up because of deep down insecurity. I looked good, but not sure if I was good.

Then, through the courageous confrontation of my then-wife, I found the beginning of sobriety on September 9, 1983, when I joined Alcoholics Anonymous. I went to meetings and met some like-minded people, but it took me several months to fully "accept" the fact that I was an alcoholic. How could someone with a Cadillac parked in a circle driveway be powerless over that substance?

But I was, and I slowly began to change. One of my "change" memories came from my new AA friend, Bill P. He was as action-oriented as I was analytical. One day, I was reviewing all the options of a quandary I was in, and Bill said to me, "You are like in a hot fire trying to understand the principles of oxidation. You've read the book—it says, 'into action,' not into thinking." He then added, "Get off your ass, make a decision, and do something, anything, even if it's wrong."

I am proud that, for once, I heard another person's constructive admonition and did take action on something that did not necessarily "look good." It was not popular, not in the majority, but it was honest and being true to the real me, which I was beginning to discover.

Also in recovery, I had a case of agoraphobia, which prevented me from being able to drive on expressways and drive or walk over bridges with water underneath. This persisted for 20 years of sobriety, and I avoided *all* of those experiences just to prevent a serious panic attack that happened whenever I tried to face those fears. That condition did pass when I took a risk to drive over a mile bridge over a river to visit someone I loved. When I truly got out of myself on that occasion, the panic passed and has never reoccurred. I am proud that I risked driving over that bridge.

Around that same time, I saw a documentary about domestic violence, and it focused primarily on verbal abuse, which triggered memories I had "buried" about how I had often spoken to my first wife. She had confronted my drinking, but we just couldn't work out our differences and had gotten divorced. She remarried. One of our children had gotten married and the first grandchild had arrived by this time, but we were enveloped in tension.

This film brought out my sorrow for the way I had treated that beautiful woman. I cried for hours. After consulting with my sponsor, I called her and made precise and detailed apologies for the way I had treated her in those awful days.

She wept profusely and thanked me for finally validating her feelings and taking responsibility to be honest about our past and giving her some closure. A few weeks later she invited me to Thanksgiving dinner with her husband and others in our family. That was in 2000 and I have gone every Thanksgiving since. And, each year on my sober anniversary, I call and thank her for the gift of confrontation that she gave me. I am proud that I took that step of personal accountability.

When I turned 80, my daughter, Molly, arranged a party for me. I was told a few days before then to arrive at 5 p.m. at a nearby banquet hall. I almost threw up—around 75 people were there, folks from Houston, Denver, Cincinnati, Northern Wisconsin, and Washington, D.C. Both of my children, all six of my grandchildren, my oldest nephew, my two former stepdaughters, friends from recovery, friends from work, former neighbors, and several folks I am privileged to sponsor attended. They roasted me pretty good, and then some of the people closest to me shared their thoughts about our friendship, how they evolved, and how they thought I had helped them. Then my daughter announced that the group all contributed to a fund for me to take a lifelong-dream train trip across Canada.

Then I was asked to speak. I stood at the podium overwhelmed with the wonder of it all, and I was keenly aware of how I used to clamor for that much attention—and that night was embarrassed by it all. I got sober, was transformed in many ways, and I am most proud of that.

I love the game of golf, which I can still play (not well, but I play). Here are lines I wrote this past summer during the British

Open that more accurately expresses my true feelings about my life and how I have evolved. I am most proud that I can feel!

Winding Down

Made a bet with my best golf buddy that

Tiger would be in contention at the Open this year.

I lost.

Yet got to see him walking the last hole

Across that Bridge, his playing partners letting him walk ahead.

Alone.

To the applause and cheers of thousands who so value the contribution he has made to this wonderful game.

My tears flowed just as I saw him dab his eyes,

And I was struck that I too am winding it down.

No fame, no fortune, but without regret for the way I have played

This game of life.

I hear no applause, no cheers, but I hear joy in my heart for the gift to just be here, winding it down for sure, but a putter in my hand and hope for another day of trying to just play the big game well!

MOLLY GORNEY

Mom of three. Wife of eighteen years. Half marathon finisher. RN who decided to go back to school in her 40s to get her degree in social work. Mom with the perfect holiday cards and Instagram posts, who was dying inside and didn't know how to stop drinking wine every night. Survivor. Someone whose insides are finally starting to match her outsides.

I know this may be hard to hear and even harder to believe. Or it may seem too simple or the thing that might actually kill you if you do it. But the thing you must do in order to stay sober is to tell the truth—to yourself and to others.

Not a version of the truth, the whole truth.

It doesn't have to be all the truths to the same person. Just have a few safe people (*human* people—dogs and cats are important, but they don't count here)—your therapist, your priest, your best friend, a sponsor, or even a stranger on the subway—that you can consistently tell your truths to as they come up each day. One at a time, truth by truth.

I know you have likely told so many lies to yourself and to others, both big and small, to be able to keep alcohol in your life. Or maybe you are drinking because of all the god-awful things you did while drinking. Or you are lying because if you say the truth that you have a problem with alcohol, you will have to give it up forever/that you are the *worst*/that [insert name here] will never love you again or that "they" will come take your kids away or never trust you alone with them again. You just know that if you tell the truth, you will literally melt into a puddle of shame and die immediately. Or the scariest thought—that if you tell the truth, you won't be able to drink like you want to or like you *need* to —again.

But I promise you, you don't ever have to drink again, and the only way to make sure that happens is if you start telling the truth.

"How does a person tell the truth?" you might ask. You can start by telling the truth to yourself. Get quiet and create space in the morning to be with yourself. This might ironically be the scariest time of your day, this time you spend with yourself. So go slow if you need to, maybe just start by actually sitting through the savasana at the end of your yoga practice. Or getting up a little earlier than everyone else in your house each morning, getting your coffee, and spending five minutes in your favorite space with your coziest blanket.

When you can stand it, maybe try writing the truth down on a piece of paper. You can burn it or tear it to shreds immediately after. But write it with your hands on an actual piece of paper to get it out of your body and *be honest*. Then maybe try speaking this truth to that human you have chosen. Do it on a walk so you don't have to look at the person while you say it or on the Marco Polo app so you won't be looking at their face and be tempted to change the version of that truth to a less truthier truth.

Start with an easy truth and keep practicing with the harder ones. Sobriety meetings are perfect places to do this because all the people there have already made themselves vulnerable by showing up and should be telling the truth. I once heard someone say that sobriety meetings are like "spiritual kindergarten," where you get to practice being the kind of truth-telling person you want to be to your loved ones with strangers who presumably don't matter.

Online meetings are fantastic for this (one of the only good things that came out of COVID-19 is that on AA Intergroup you can literally find hundreds of online AA meetings, 24 hours a day, in all the languages you can think of). You can come to the meeting with your camera off, to a meeting in a different country than your own, with a different name, and even use a voice modifier if you feel so inclined to tell your truth.

I promise it won't kill you. In fact, I promise it will be thing that actually might save you.

"What if the truth doesn't come out, or I don't even know how to tell the truth?"

If you sit long enough and allow enough space for it, it will come. Some days it will keep coming, even when you try to stop it, like the dry heaves the day after you drank a bottle and a half of wine, when you promised yourself this time you would just have two glasses. And some days it will surprise you.

I heard a perfect metaphor for this in yet another sobriety meeting, because that is where all the best things are said. Someone said they had a friend who was in a terrible car accident that had left him with tiny shards of glass embedded all over his body—so many pieces of glass that the surgeons couldn't remove them all.

Years after the accident, little slivers of glass would randomly poke through his skin when this person least expected it, and the person at the meeting likened it to the unexpected painful moments that can happen in sobriety. Those painful pieces of glass breaking through your skin will feel like the truths you must tell some days—especially those truths that you tucked into the deepest parts of your being so that no one could ever find them. You might have even forgotten that they happened as a form of self-protection, as a form of sheer survival.

These truths are the ones that need to come out most of all, whether they seem big or small to you now, because they are the ones that are rotting away at the essence of your soul, perhaps without your even realizing it. Like the time you drove your kids home from soccer while it was still daylight, and you were so inebriated you had to squint with one eye open in order to get home. Or the time you breastfed your baby in the middle of the night when you knew you had one too many glasses of wine, but you just wanted the baby to stop crying. Maybe the time you snuck away to the store to replace the empty wine bottle before your partner got home, so he wouldn't know how much you had, and you could keep drinking. Or maybe the truths have nothing to do with alcohol—like the seething resentment you feel towards your partner every night while he sits comfortably in his chair scrolling his iPhone while you cook dinner and manage the kids, or the abortion you had in college that only you and your then-boyfriend know about, or all the things you want to say to your mom who constantly makes passive-aggressive remarks about your weight or the way you raise your kids.

These resentments, these truths that you are keep inside, are keeping you stuck. They are keeping you in a cycle that is so painful that you feel like you have no choice but to have one or four glasses of wine every night to take the edge off, so you don't go insane.

Start to tell these truths, and you start to heal. It won't be easy, but let's be honest. Managing the hangovers, parenting, and going to work every day with that dull headache and the slight twinge of nausea aren't easy, either. So maybe, just for today, try another way and see how it goes.

Once you start telling the truth and living a life of integrity, you will find it a little easier to say "no" to that glass of wine. I promise. Self-esteem comes from doing esteemable acts. If you slip and drink the wine, that's okay. Tell that truth in a meeting or to someone you trust, dust yourself off, and start again. As one of my very wise teachers, Laura McKowen, says, push off from here.

You can do this, you can stop drinking, you can save your own life. And you can start by telling the truth.

NATALIE AUSTIN

Holistic recovery coach. Yoga and meditation teacher. Meeting leader at The Luckiest Club. Mama to three. Nanny to three. Lover of all things woo. Truth teller. Alchemist. Teetotaler. Waking up hangover-free will never, ever get old for me.

Sometimes it feels like it has been 10 minutes and sometimes it feels like it has been 10 years since I decided to remove alcohol from my life. August 2015 was when I had my last drink, and these years have been full of highs, lows, and everything in between. But one thing I know for certain is that this life would be so damn different if I had not put the booze down.

I would most certainly not own my own home. I would most certainly not be a successful, holistic recovery and wellness coach, yoga teacher, meditation teacher, or own and create blends for my essential oil business.

I would not have had the wherewithal to leave relationships that no longer served me. I would not have been able to be fully present for my kids, grandkids, family, and friends. I would not have been able to unpack much of the trauma and dis-ease that had led me to a place of needing to numb out, to dissociate from myself and my body (and my life, honestly), and I would not have had the presence of mind to understand myself and begin to self-regulate and get my nervous system back on track. And I know more than anything, that I would not be head-over-heels in love with myself and this big, beautiful, delicious life, the way that I am today.

When I gave up drinking, I did not—to the outside world—look like I had much of an issue. I would have considered myself a high-functioning drinker. I was successful, was a mama, was in a great relationship, and had a big circle of friends with whom I partied all of the time. As a matter of fact, we all fit that same mold of drinking, having fun, and living it up—work hard, play hard—but it got to the point for me that one was too many, and 10 was never enough.

I stopped having an off-switch or a way to just have one. It became a worrisome venture when I had that first drink—I never really knew if I was going to black out or say something stupid, or even worse, do something stupid when I was drinking. It always seemed to end up as a bit of a crap shoot as to the outcome of the events of my drinking.

My life that was so rooted in shame, disappointment, and disdain for myself that I could not control my drinking; resentment for needing to hide what I was really going through; and anger for all of the things that made me feel the need to constantly drink.

Once I finally removed alcohol, I knew I needed to find a practice of some kind to help get me through the ups and downs of recovery. So I decided to find a yoga studio and see if that would calm my monkey mind. I had always been the girl who went to lunchtime boot camp classes to punish myself for being hungover again—always doing the more ego-based workouts instead of something that would be more nourishing for my mind, body, and spirit.

I found more in yoga than I could have ever expected. I found a moving meditation—a way to quiet my monkey mind, to really just arrive and be in my body, while also getting a pretty awesome workout. I had never experienced the ease of self that I found in yoga. I had never experienced the ability to just arrive into my body, focus on my breath, focus on the next pose, and really push myself to stay, to breathe, and to just be.

Some days, I would practice yoga twice, as I just could not get enough of how it made me feel, of how it helped me show up, of how it brought so much ease to my usually intense brain, body, and emotions. I also found a community, which helped me stay connected to the practice and also to myself.

I credit much of my success in recovery to building a toolbox of tangible and intangible items as I started down the road of removing alcohol and creating a life I did not need to numb or escape from. Tangible tools are physical items or practices you can use to aid in your sobriety, while intangible tools are more abstract concepts or practices that can help support your emotional and mental well-being.

My favorite tangible tools are essential oils, crystals, and smudging with sage, palo santo and copal. Also one of the most magical parts of sobriety is experiencing my early mornings. They certainly did not exist when I was drinking, but now they are the very favorite part of my day. Rise before the sun, coffee, meditation, music, read, writing, and prepping for the day. I love that it can be as in depth or minimal as it is a process and a practice.

Just being with myself in the early morning hours is such a gift —it is a grounding practice that creates a solid foundation, keeps me in my body, and sets me up for a calmer way of being throughout my day. I can tell a difference in the mornings when I do not make time for this practice—I feel a palpable difference throughout my day.

Another practice that consistently helps me is really leaning into my spirituality and creating an ongoing spiritual practice. A spiritual practice can take many different forms, depending on the individual and his or her beliefs. Generally speaking, a spiritual practice involves regular activities or rituals that are designed to deepen our connection with a higher power, with our own inner self or the divine.

My spiritual practice includes yoga asana, which refers to the physical postures or positions practiced in yoga and can feel like a moving-breath meditation, as I spoke about earlier. Meditation/mindfulness and quieting the mind to focus on the present moment to become more aware of my thoughts, feelings, and surroundings, and just being able to pause and be with my breath is an anchor I can create throughout my day.

My daily rituals also include lighting sage and smudging my home, lighting candles, pulling a tarot card, and reading about the moon cycle and astrology. Having a clear understanding of these cycles helps me unpack some of the intense or softening feelings that show up. To consistently connect with something greater than myself feels so nourishing to my nervous system and creates deep ease for me to manage the ups and downs of being human.

Through all of the tools, rituals, processes, and practices I have created and continue to embody, I have really learned how to embrace being human—to embrace the light and the dark, to embrace the idea of impermanence and that we are all just doing our very best. As the incredible, spiritual teacher Ram Dass says, "We are all just walking each other home."

TAMMI SALAS

Sober. Dignified. Creative. Woman. Former wine bar owner, PTA president, people pleaser and dinner party thrower.

Early in my sobriety, I figured out that in order to stay the course without drinking, I needed some accountability or routine to help keep me sober for the day. Not the week. Not the month. Not the year. Just for the 24 hours directly in front of me.

Routines are hardwired for me. As a former legal secretary, a Virgo, and a type 2w1 on the Enneagram (the one being very strong), routines make me feel safe. I find comfort in knowing the next thing to do and just doing it. I realized I had to cut out some of the unknown in my day and create a foundation for my sobriety to rest on. It wasn't easy, and I definitely learned a lot along the way.

The year before I got sober, I started an accountability practice inspired by artist Lisa Congdon. You see, Lisa liked to embark on yearlong daily projects, write about them, share them publicly on social media to help keep her accountable, and, in some instances, she would publish the project in a book when she was done. Everything about this sparked something inside of me.

On January 1, 2014, I embarked on my own accountability

project of creating art every day in a journal and sharing my process on my blog and social media. This was over nine years ago, during the last year of my drinking—which was the worst year of my drinking, accompanied by repetitive, soul-crushing hangovers.

Every morning, I woke up and did the fake sober, pretending I didn't feel like hell and frantically trying to put together what had happened the night before. How did it end? Did I embarrass myself? Do I have any bruises or injuries?

As a blackout drinker, this is what I like to refer to as Sober C.S.I.— you know, engaging in sober investigative activities to piece together the night before and look for clues to inform me about my behavior.

How was my car parked?

Where was my purse?

Who did I text?

Why was I still dressed, but my shoes were nowhere to be found?

Was my husband mad at me?

You know, Sober C.S.I.

On January 1, 2014, I woke up with a splitting-headache hangover, sat down at my kitchen table with a brand new journal, and wrote in colored pencil the word: Acceptance. It was my word for the year, and I embellished it with a few swirls. Nothing fancy. It was a start.

I continued this practice every day that year. It was a working meditation. It gave me a lot of time to think about my life and why I was so unhappy.

At the end of 2014, on New Year's Eve, I illustrated a quote credited to Eleanor Roosevelt that said, "Happiness is the byproduct of a well-lived life."

I sat at my kitchen table and cried like I had never cried before. The year had been so hard, my drinking was beyond out of hand, and my health was deteriorating.

I was so proud for keeping my word to myself with this journal project, because up until that morning, I realized I had been betraying myself for so long that even I didn't believe me. Finishing this project felt like a major personal victory.

I was embarrassed to be so proud, so I kept my feelings to myself, but I quickly decided that I would keep going with the project for the coming year.

It would take me another 33 days until I would have my last drink, on Groundhog Day 2015. I haven't had a drink since.

I continue making art in some, way, shape, or form every day. It is my medicine, my church, and my way of showing up in the world now. It solidifies something in me that I don't even fully understand. It calms my central nervous system and reminds me that I have the power and choice to create beauty in my own life.

I started moving my body.

I stopped wearing contact lenses.

I quit dyeing my hair.

I quit drinking coffee.

I started drinking tea.

I attended 12-step meetings.

I got a sponsor and worked the 12 steps.

I got up early every morning to read books by spiritual teachers.

I joined sober communities.

I made new friends.

Creativity is a practice, and it helped save me from myself. I still create something every day—a list using my own handwriting (my personal font!), or a simple watercolor, collage or sketch. I create with my fashion and style, my adornment, and how I decorate my home. I create beautiful meals, set a simple table, arrange flowers, and ritualize my morning tea pours.

I pick a song when I wake up and use it as my theme song for the day. I organize my bookshelves to be aesthetically pleasing and spray paint tumbleweeds to hang from my ceiling just because I can. I wear red lipstick because it makes me happy and keep a logbook to jot down my daily doings so that I can remember this beautiful life I've created in sobriety.

I like creating meaning out of my rituals and routines.

I like the metaphor for life that art generously allows.

I like that nothing has to be perfect and that perfect is actually pretty boring.

I like creating beauty from nothing.

Once I stopped drinking, I quickly realized I had a god-sized hole inside of me that needed to be filled. Since I could no longer fill it with booze, I decided to go back to college at 44 years old and major in art. The discipline, the structure, and all the basic math (oy vey!) gave me purpose and direction for those first few years of sobriety.

Attending college, going to sobriety support meetings, daily art making, following spiritual practices, and attending workshops and therapy have helped me navigate this alcohol-free journey over the years.

My alcohol problem presented me with a portal through which I could pass so I could start creating a beautiful life that I no longer wanted to escape from. I am the architect of my own life, and I get to create my happily ever after. I had to change the way I was doing things so that, in turn, my life could change. I'm so grateful I've had this chance.

I like to say I create my own fun in sobriety. And I want you to know that you can, too.

ANDI L.K.

Parent of three, grad student, autistic, queer.

Removing alcohol from my life allowed me to gain clarity into my true purpose and calling in the world. I am currently studying to be a clinical mental health counselor, focusing on trauma, grief, and addiction. My greatest achievement has been the threefold process of listening to my intuition, taking action to pursue my goals, and succeeding in my program of study — none of which would have happened while alcohol was still playing a significant role in my life.

When I was drinking alcohol regularly, I was intentionally trying to drown out and ignore my inner knowledge and numb, painful feelings around family member illnesses and deaths, social and relational conflict, and work issues. I had no idea what I really wanted to do or be "when I grew up."

Once I became a parent, I expected my life to spontaneously fill to the brim with meaning to the extent that I wouldn't need to worry about anything else. While my children have brought immense meaning, as well as both joys and challenges, I still felt a tiny, nagging sensation of needing to do something more. This fact itself contributed to my drinking as I tried to cover feelings of guilt around thinking I didn't appreciate my role as a mom enough.

After I stopped using alcohol for the final time, I experienced the overwhelming rush of "all the feelings," that is familiar to so many folks in early recovery. Over the next few months, as the intensity of those emotions began to settle into a smoother, more regulated pattern, that quiet voice telling me to do something else in my life steadily grew louder.

Having spent the previous 18 years ignoring my intuition, I was still hesitant and afraid of what that voice was saying. Then, one day in a sobriety support meeting, the leader read from Steven Pressfield's *The War of Art*, including the quote, "The more scared we are of a work or calling, the more sure we can be that we have to do it."

I knew immediately that I needed to really listen to and follow the voice of intuition telling me to become a death doula (an end-of-life guide who provides informational and emotional support). I followed through on my intuition and enrolled in a certificate course, where I learned about logistical support for folks at the end of life, and also about the processes of anticipatory and complex grief.

An even deeper truth began to surface for me that I was being called to use my past experiences of grief to offer compassion and support to others on their grief journeys, and I began taking further action to pursue grief counselor training at the master's level.

Throughout these stages of embracing my inner knowledge more and more deeply, I was also continuing to learn about connections between addiction and trauma and other mental health concerns. As I continue pursuing my intuition and navigating my new educational and professional path, I am repeatedly rewarded for listening to my heart by discovering additional layers of truth and guidance toward fulfillment. Taking steps to follow these new insights has built my confidence and trust in myself and my ability to know what is good for me, instead of using alcohol to numb the inner conflict of doing whatever *others* thought was good for me.

At this time, I am approaching the halfway point of my coursework and have been invited to join the honor society for counseling students and professionals. While I am often exhausted, I am no longer making myself more tired and sick on a daily basis by consuming alcohol. I am able to focus on intense emotionally and mentally challenging work during the day, because I am not hungover, as well as in the evenings, because I'm not spending my limited free time drinking.

Furthermore, between my own personal therapy and the knowledge I'm gaining through my studies, I am actually a much better parent to my three kids. Simply not drinking made a hugely positive impact in my ability to parent attentively and gently. By taking these additional steps of listening to my intuition, I believe I am setting a very different example, which hopefully will break the cycle of intergenerational trauma and substance use into which I was born.

I am certainly not a perfect parent, but my kids get to see me trying to do better and apologizing when I make mistakes. They see me being present and involved instead of mentally checked out. And they see me working hard to pursue a new dream. If they learn anything from me, I hope they grow up knowing it is never too late to change directions and choose a new, more fulfilling path.

Sometimes I still can't quite believe I am actually "doing the thing" and progressing steadily through my studies. My past self, who was constantly in avoidance and survival mode, would have laughed out loud at the idea that I could ever help someone else with their mental health concerns. I had been depressed, anxious, and self-medicating for nearly twenty years before finally achieving sustained sobriety.

While I continue to work on managing my own mental health with therapy and medication, I have the grounded clarity of knowing that my experiences can be useful to others. I trust that I can empathize deeply with folks who are in a place of pain and darkness, and I can gently and compassionately, without judgment, walk alongside others in their healing journeys as my support community has done for me.

ANDREA MURPHY

Boy and dog mom. Corporate compliance officer. Lover of learning, connection, and growth. Alcohol was my best friend, until it wasn't, and no one knew the extent of my drinking. I have given up one thing (alcohol) and gotten everything in return.

My attempts to abstain from alcohol and try to moderate my drinking started in earnest in my late 30s after I had children, although I knew as early as age 33 that I likely had an issue with alcohol. And by issue, I mean that alcohol held a prominent role and absorbed a significant amount of time in my daily life.

This caused some concern because of the alcohol abuse that had occurred in my family during my childhood and beyond. I say, "issue" rather than problem, because I didn't start to see alcohol as problematic and detrimental until much later; mainly because I would not accept that my beloved wine and martinis could possibly be problematic, even though I frequently experienced negative effects during and after drinking.

The negative effects included arguments that escalated in ways that would likely not have happened if I had not been drinking (and not even being able to figure out later why I got so upset in the first place), hangovers, risky behavior, and blackouts. Even if I didn't have a full-blown hangover, I often felt less than 100 percent healthy like I did on days that I didn't drink.

Then my drinking became a daily event, and I forgot what it was like to ever feel 100 percent healthy. I believed because I was "healthy" otherwise—eating well, exercising, and drinking tons of water—that the bad effects of alcohol were minimal for me. This wasn't true, of course, but I needed to believe this. Otherwise I would have had to take a serious look at my "best friend," alcohol.

My life is self-made. I came from a long line of family members who did not have the resources or the desire to further their education or pursue a career. From a young age, I knew that I needed and wanted to get out of my rural town in Kentucky and pursue college and a career. I could do those things by working full time and putting myself through college, paying for nearly everything that I had from the time I was 16 to today at 51.

Being someone who is highly motivated and driven, I couldn't understand why I struggled so much with moderating my drinking. This didn't make sense to me because my life had no other part where I felt "unable" to do something. My career was going well, I ran a marathon, I had two kids under the age of four, and I was promoted to a great position in my company by the time I was 39.

I powered through sleepless nights during the first few years of motherhood and delivered on work deadlines, worked out, and stayed socially active. I also daily pursued alcohol and the "mommy wine culture" at this point. I look back and am amazed at the resilience of the human body and mind at powering through so much—especially for women who work full time and manage the responsibilities of young children and a household. All while drinking alcohol/ethanol daily. After being alcohol-free for a significant time, I say now that I managed to accomplish a lot with one arm (or both) tied behind my back.

At 42, I woke up one morning and realized that something had to change. My tolerance level for alcohol was rising, and I knew too much about the harmful effects of alcohol to ignore the discrepancy between what the surgeon general states is a "safe" amount of alcohol for women and the amount I was regularly consuming. The cognitive dissonance was making me very uncomfortable, and I started, in earnest, to become alcohol-free.

However, I didn't really want to give up alcohol yet. I felt deprived and like I was "missing out." I also believed that the only way I could truly relax was to have a drink. Now, mind you, this is the marketing message of the multi-billion-dollar alcohol industry: "Drinking makes you relax, have fun, be sexier, super-human." All a lie, as it turns out, but I still believed that message at this point.

I white-knuckled through six months of not drinking. It was difficult, but my mind became clear for the first time in years. My body felt better. My eyes were clear and bright again. And yet, I still struggled to believe that life could be truly better without alcohol.

I had no friends or people surrounding me who were alcohol-free. My profession encourages drinking and provided unlimited amounts of alcohol at meetings, making it difficult to abstain when traveling for work—not to mention the questions we get when we don't drink.

No one asks why you don't smoke, do pot, or snort cocaine, but if you don't drink, watch out, here comes the interrogation. Interestingly, alcohol does more damage and causes more deaths than smoking and other illicit drugs combined now, according to addictioncenter.com, but very few people realize this until they take a closer look at what alcohol really is and what it does to those who drink it on a regular basis.

I spent another seven years fighting the moderation battle. Moderation simply did not work for me. I didn't understand it. How could I not get control of this thing?

Then I found a resource that changed, and likely saved, my life: *This Naked Mind* by Annie Grace. When I read this book, I was literally stunned at how much I did not understand about the vicious cycle of physical and mental effects that alcohol causes, even on days when you don't drink.

The way this book scientifically explained this started to

change how I viewed alcohol and my response to it. Where I once felt shame at not being able to control my drinking, I now understood why I couldn't. I also could no longer argue that alcohol had any positive attributes. It is a poison, and it destroys what it touches.

Something in me shifted once I understood that, and suddenly I was able to give up alcohol and feel liberated and joyful about it. While it took me years to give up alcohol, once I did, I found it relatively easy to stay sober. I found a group of amazing people who are on a similar journey within The Luckiest Club (TLC), founded by Laura McKowen.

Even though I no longer want alcohol in my life, our culture makes it challenging to stay sober. Being involved with a group of people with the same goals and who support each other has helped me through the tough moments. This has also brought amazing resources into my life, along with significant connections and friendships.

The stigma around abstaining from alcohol and what that means is changing. "Are you an alcoholic?" people often ask. But that's the wrong question in my opinion. The better question is "Is alcohol serving you and improving your life, or are you serving alcohol and suffering detrimental effects?"

No one has to reach a rock bottom to make a change. I believe stopping the elevator and getting off before it hits the ground is a much better choice.

ANGIE CHAPLIN

Mindful Leadership teacher, consultant, and speaker grounded in integrity, curiosity, clarity, connection, and love. Generator, Enneagram 7w8, yogi. Boy mom of two emerging adults and one dog in Iowa City. Living, loving, and leading a sober life of my own design since Groundhog Day 2020.

I was 40 days into my sober journey when the COVID-19 lockdown halted the in-person outpatient services that had become the building blocks for my newfound sobriety. Living alone, isolated from friends and family, I reached a turning point.

Despite life-threatening consequences, falling back into old drinking patterns seemed like the easy route, especially when the rest of the world, as I knew it, was turning to alcohol to cope with what would become a global pandemic.

I consciously chose a different road that was not only less traveled but also non-existent. With a background in organizational culture, strategy, and leadership, I knew enough about myself to realize I needed more actionable tools than what 12-step programs offered. Brainstorming any possible resources that could help me keep moving forward on my journey, I remembered a values identification and alignment exercise from graduate school.

The Leadership Challenge by authors Jim Kouzes and Barry Posner was the first textbook in the first module of Seton Hall University's Master of Arts program in strategic communication and leadership (MASCL). The book had such a significant impact on me that I had continued my studies to achieve certified master status for *The Leadership Challenge.* But that had been more than a decade earlier, and years of alcohol use had taken my life in very different directions.

Feeling like a sober fish out of water and trying to stay afloat from self-deprecating thoughts about losing my own leadership skills, I dug through boxes of old textbooks and materials to find *The Leadership Challenge.* Sitting alone at my kitchen table, I recreated the values exercise and landed on an epiphany that was even more powerful than when I'd experienced it the first time, 15 years earlier.

Back then, I had poured myself into various roles—partner, mother, friend, daughter, professional, volunteer, leader—and had little left for myself.

And during the pandemic, my life was similar—I had lost touch with who I was. Values could guide me back to myself in mind, body, and spirit.

Looking at the words on the values cards that were part of the exercise—growth, connection, wellbeing, gratitude, and love—I made a commitment. As I had learned as a grad school student, then taught as a faculty member, aligning my actions with those words would integrate behaviors that represented the truest, most beautiful version of who I was—to lead me forward in freedom from alcohol. I made a commitment to act with authenticity by staying grounded in my values.

Values became the compass I used to set goals, make decisions, and take action. When faced with choices on how to spend my time, money, and energy (our most valuable currency), the questions include, "How does _____ align with my values?" or "How does _____ align with creating a life of my own design?"

Letting values lead the way doesn't mean I ignore other important and realistic factors in decision-making or refuse to seek others' advice. It does mean that I'm mindful about choosing what is right based on my values, the information I have available, and my intuition. At times, living into my values meant having to make painful decisions, like choosing to end a relationship, leaving a lucrative job, or turning down opportunities that didn't feel right.

I have learned that even when things are going well at home, at work, or in life, when something feels off, it's time for a values check-in. Authors and experts recommend values-based systems, habits, and leadership styles—from Brené Brown in several of best-selling books, most recently, *Atlas of the Heart*, to James Clear in *Atomic Habits*.

Living a sober life is hard. And, as encouraged by author Glennon Doyle in *Untamed*, we can do hard things. I have learned that doing hard things is easier when I have a clear understanding of my values, the direction they are pointing me toward, and connection with people willing to walk the talk beside me.

Choosing to lean into my values to lead me away from alcohol was the best decision I've ever made.

BEN OWENS

Sober for eight-plus years. Single dad of twin seven-year-old girls. Loves golf, sports, reading, and gardening. I have a reverse bachelor's degree in how to live. Overthinker, shy, insecure, fearful, emotional, and alone. Kind, hilarious, assertive, balanced, outgoing, loyal, intelligent, friendly, and loved. History nerd. I have grit; you do too.

For me maintaining sobriety was initially a live-or-die situation. Medical issues landed me in the hospital yet again: liver failure, kidney failure, yada, yada, yada.

A priest read my last rites, and I wasn't expected to make it through the night. I did, and upon waking, was told if I drank again, I would die. I had developed cirrhosis after 20 years of struggling, four detoxes, facilities, etc.

This was the one time something stuck, thank God. I walked into my first AA meeting around at 6:30 in the morning to a smoke-filled room. I picked it because I could smoke.

The first two to three years of my sobriety, I relied on meetings upon meetings, morning lunch, evening. I probably overdid it, to be honest, but I was desperate, of course, like we always are. In hindsight, I know I could have made some better decisions in sobriety. I could have found a sponsor or mentor and worked my steps sooner. I waited for three years.

The people in that first meeting I went to turned out to be my "group," and we relied heavily on each other. We also did not want to let each other down, so there was a natural, unforced sense of accountability.

I continued to go to meetings three to four times a week and on Saturdays until about six years in when COVID-19 hit. My regular meeting disbanded, but as I learned early in sobriety, this is a new life—I had to learn how to re-navigate my way through.

Today I don't have to even think about not drinking or staying sober. The only way I got here was through the support I had sought and built, consistency, the Big Guy upstairs, and a desire to stay sober.

One of the most valuable and important things I have learned on this journey is that it is my fault 99.9 percent of the time when something goes wrong in my life. Another is that it is okay, if not essential, to let go of control. For me, that meant to let go and let God run the show.

That was a tough one to swallow. I was raised Catholic and I'm proud to a fault. This concept took me about five-plus years to embrace fully. It was one of the best choices I've ever made. I'm no longer in control of everyone and everything around me. I credit God and the village for my sobriety. I tried for 20 years by myself; not the smartest plan.

In my experience, there was no quick fix. It takes time to totally relearn how to think and to relearn how to behave. Without booze in my hand, what would I do at weddings, parties, and concerts? What would I tell people? They know me as the party guy. *What if … ? What now?*

These questions are pretty universal for newly sober individuals. The answer was: It will work itself out. A line in the AA meeting readings says, "You will intuitively know how to handle situations."

It's true. One of the things I could have done better early on is not stress about the future. I was told not to a million times, but it was difficult for me to grasp. I compensated by working out too often and overdoing most things in my life.

I had to substitute one addiction for another, so exercise took over, and when that wasn't doing it, I started gambling. I needed the dopamine hit. I, of course, can see these things in hindsight, and it is so clear to me what I was chasing. At the time, however, I was so focused on my sobriety that I wasn't stepping back to look at myself and see how I was doing. I was fortunate that I had a home group and AA friends to share this with.

I forced myself to be honest about my shortcomings in sobriety. I was convinced that sobriety automatically equaled perfect behavior and no roadblocks. It didn't, but there are basically pebbles compared to boulders and a three-car pile-up that the problems were when I was drinking.

Being able to share and to be 100 percent open and honest with a person or a group was key for me. When I could look at someone and know they had felt the same shame, the same anger, same hurts, disappointments, humiliations, and anxiety as I had and know there was no judgment of any kind, that was life changing. I only found complete empathy because I was not alone. We've all done the same embarrassing things, and ruined relationships.

A peace came that I did not expect. It comes when you realize that you are not alone. You were never alone, you just decided to isolate yourself and live in a make-believe fairyland in your head. I won the Masters' numerous times when I was drunk late at night —fairytale land! But in real life it was incredibly reassuring that I was not alone.

Since COVID–19, my AA meeting attendance has gone down. Not because I don't think I need it, or it is less valuable, but because my home group was primarily comprised of older individuals with many years of sobriety. COVID–19 drove many of them to online meetings.

I like to gather with others physically. I get more out of it, but that is just me. I am certain that I will attend meetings for life. I don't necessarily agree with all aspects of AA, but I have learned to take what works for me and leave the rest. If I feel off or easily agitated, I quickly identify what is going on with me.

Self-awareness is one of the strongest defenses against the drive to drink. If I'm not mindful, I can easily get too high or too low or too happy or too sad. It doesn't matter which emotion presents itself; they are all dangerous. A cliché that is 1,000 percent correct: Everything in moderation.

I had to learn how to moderate myself emotionally. It is as simple as, "Be a good person.". My dad says, "Don't be a dick." If I can manage to do the right thing and to be honest with others and myself, open, consistent, and let God run the show, maintaining my sobriety is pretty simple. It was a lot of work to get here, and I have only scratched the surface of sobriety.

Since I've been sober I have:

Had two amazing, twin girls.

Hung out with Charles Barkley, Eddie Vedder, Theo Eppstein, Chris Chelios, and Dennis Rodman for three hours before and after a Pearl Jam show at Wrigley—Eddie Vedder told me I have a "nice physique." 😊

Had a hole in one.

Been in major motion picture with Leo and De Niro.

Taught high school history.

Survived a pandemic.

Coached my girls' soccer team.

Was at Game Six at Wrigley when the Cubs beat the Dodgers to go to the World Series for the first time in 108 years!

Traveled all over.

I'm still alive.

CARRIE MAY

Highly functional alcoholic. Daily drinker sobriety advocate. Founder of non-profit Chicago AF. Volunteer sobriety event organizer hosting monthly social activities, which are intentionally inclusive of everyone. Founder of Brave Recovery Coaching Practice hosts sobriety hiking retreats. Mission to normalize sobriety and advance the NA movement. Emergency department nurse practitioner.

My greatest personal achievement in my sobriety has been getting to a point where I could recover out loud. This took over four years.

When I entered sobriety, I was filled with *so* much shame. I'm not honestly sure what was worse. The mom shame vs. the medical provider shame. I entered sobriety on April 4, 2016. This was before modern recovery. No one openly talked about drinking back then and definitely not anyone I knew. You were either an alcoholic or you were not. The term gray-area drinking did not exist. Not that it mattered; I was not a gray-area drinker. I was completely addicted to alcohol.

My whole adult life, I drank. It was not problematic until a few years before I stopped. My switch for the most part had remained intact. As a lifetime high achiever, mother of two, and nurse practitioner, I simply started drinking more after work. That's it. No major life event, no tragedy. The increase was gradual.

I knew when my switch flipped. But I could not talk about it. My husband tried to talk to me. He tried everything. I couldn't talk about it because that would mean I had a problem. And if I had a problem, I would have to stop. Also, I could not deal with being an alcoholic. Not that—anything but that. Not deliberate thinking, just engrained thinking.

When the crossroads inevitably came, I chose my family over the option to continue drinking. I had to choose one or the other. Although people will say, "You have to get sober for yourself," I got sober for my children and husband. Whatever your motive is at the beginning, do it. It doesn't matter. Eventually I was sober for myself, but that took time.

My early recovery (first three years) was not easy. I wish I could say it was. I struggled hard with shame, especially since I was a nurse practitioner, and an unwritten code of disdain exists in the medical community against those that have alcohol use disorder. I know it firsthand because I experienced it every day.

The reason I struggled so hard is because the stigma is real. Although we are making strides with the alcohol-free movement changing societal perceptions, the medical community is lagging. When I saw my PCP for a follow-up visit after treatment for an unrelated reason (horrified that the records were even sent to her), she told me I would relapse. Zero compassion. This was a provider I had specifically chosen as I watched her train.

Later, I asked my addiction specialist if she could please remove "alcohol abuse" from my medical diagnoses. I know that once you are labeled, you are labeled forever. Period. She did not. My next PCP kindly removed it for me. Sigh of relief. Now I could see a provider without the "A" word attached to name from the moment you meet me.

As I continued on my sobriety journey, my confidence grew. I started to feel comfortable in my own skin and mentored other women. I started seeking new opportunities to meet other people in recovery and create spaces for sober community. One of my proudest personal accomplishments is that despite the shame, stigma, and fear I felt, I pushed through. Hard. And I made it to the other side. The magic of long-term sobriety.

During the pandemic, I became a certified recovery coach. Virtually meeting and training with fellow coaches internationally encouraged me to start thinking outside of my suburbia box. My sobriety has exploded my nuclear world. Sobriety enables me to connect with people from all over the world with backgrounds from different industries and exposes me to new opportunities.

For instance, next week I am meeting a friend from an Instagram sober community from Spain at a launch party for a new sober magazine in New York City. This year I got to attend a She Recovers event in Miami with 600 women and The Luckiest Club in Chicago.

I have ideas that are bigger than my wildest dreams, like launching my own coaching business, Brave, and hosting all-inclusive hiking sobriety retreats with private chefs and yogis in places like Asheville, Sedona, Yosemite, and Zion. And these ideas have all become realities. I am able to gently and kindly help other women work on their own acceptance and confidence in sobriety.

I have the gift of being a leader whose passion, motivation, and enthusiasm started a non-profit sober community, Chicago AF, in the Chicago area. This community leads free, weekly online meetings, hosts a group chat, offers a mentor program, and plans monthly events. Those meetups went from small-scale meetups to hosting Chicago's first No Booze Cruise and planning Chicago's first NA tasting events.

I have spoken and written articles about my story—a story that once devastated me and brought me to my knees; a story that caused me to not be able to speak and cry at recovery meeting tables for over a year. A story that *could not* be *my* story. A story that is probably your story, too.

My greatest achievement, however, is being brave enough to recover out loud—to be the person others can feel comfortable asking for help. One of my colleagues in the emergency department recently asked if she could talk to me at work. She sat down and started, "I think I have a problem with my drinking, and X said I should talk to you." That, right there, is everything to me.

I am brave enough.

The essence of my maintaining my sobriety boils down to consistent, daily commitment. At my deepest core, I know I am only one drink away from reentering my previous addiction. I hold my sobriety in the highest regard, protect it at all costs, and surround myself with others in recovery.

I started attending AA the very morning after I got out of treatment. Although AA is the last room I ever wanted to step into, it has been the greatest gift of my entire life. AA not only gave me the tools to stay sober, it continues to give me guidance for living.

I am so grateful that my sobriety is grounded in the foundation of AA. Nothing is like the vulnerability, mutual respect, and connection of sitting in a room with others in recovery. I feel the tears sprouting as I sit, let my guard down, listen, and focus on my sobriety.

Besides attending recovery meetings, I also lead them. This accountability to others helps me stay accountable to myself. Consistent service work is key to maintaining my sobriety. For more than three years, I co-led a weekly sobriety meeting at the treatment center I attended. It took time to build up the confidence to do this, but it was extremely important to me to give back and inspire hope to those actively walking the same path I did. I have since transitioned my service work into taking recovery meetings to Cook County Jail.

Mentoring, sponsoring, and coaching others in sobriety constantly fuels my excitement for sobriety. I love working with newbies, to watch them open up, grow, and eventually own their sobriety. It is an honor for me to work with others. Honesty, vulnerability, shared experiences, and actively listening is the greatest gift we can give each other.

My relationship with my children is now authentic, deep and rich. My daughter hated my guts at age 11 and taped notes to my box of wine asking me to please stop drinking. Today, she is my biggest cheerleader. My son does not remember a time when I drank. My relationship with my husband has repaired, and he fully supports me and my sobriety endeavors.

Openly discussing my sobriety with my children from the beginning has been one of the best decisions I have ever made. Getting sober and setting the tone that we share openly about both the drinking and recovery in my family has been paramount to repairing my relationships.

Setting and upholding boundaries has been integral to my sobriety, too. If I feel overly anxious about attending an event, I don't go. If I want to leave early, I leave. To this day, with more than six years of continuous sobriety, I do not like to be around alcohol. Period. It makes me feel uncomfortable, and I am at peace with that. I actually hope that feeling never leaves me.

Utilizing healthy coping skills each day helps me stay sober. My favorite tools are quiet time and sleeping. Quieting my mind is essential to my sanity, especially with the chaotic energy of working as a nurse practitioner in an emergency department and raising two active teenagers. When I really need to tap out, I lay down or go to sleep. I pull the blanket up over my head at any time of day. This signals to my family that I need a time out.

Maintaining my sobriety also looks like staying in constant connection with my friends in recovery. Checking in on them, meeting face-to-face, and picking up the phone to hear their voices. It also requires my being honest about how I am doing. Rather than saying, "Everything is okay," I talk about how I really am. Sobriety has taught me that I need to talk about it—whatever it may be.

Finding my tribe took some time and a lot of effort. I knew I needed more connection than my recovery meetings, so I put myself out there again and again. I tried various attempts to meet others that flopped, but I did not give up. The pandemic and the era of online meetings enabled me to connect with others in a way that did not exist before. This was the game changer and allowed me to find my people.

Probably my best overall advice to maintaining my sobriety is that I "say it out loud." If I entertain the thought of a drink, I tell someone—immediately and regardless of the reason. The moment I share the words, "I feel like taking a drink," the thought loses its power. I do not allow drinking thoughts to stay in my head.

JBRO BROWN

I hold a Ph.D. in seeking comfort, yet ironically, it makes me miserable. To achieve one of my most significant milestones in sobriety, creating the Pandemic Sober Squad, I had to push past the boundaries of my comfort zone, connecting and healing in the process.

The Pandemic Sober Squad Camp's inaugural photo will always be a part of my Facebook page. In the snap, we all look orderly and happy, like a school picture. Our slogan summarizes it perfectly: "Come Be Awkward With Us." When I see those smiling faces in the image, I'm sent back to April 2022.

I created the Pandemic Sober Squad (PSS) in May 2020, that momentous pandemic spring. It all started with Laura McKowen and the Luckiest Club. At that first official TLC meeting, some of us newly nutty sober folks shared in the chat how weird it was to get sober during the pandemic. I wrote, "We should be called the Pandemic Sober Squad." Amidst the unknown, a concept was born out of fuzzy brains, messy emotions, and people staring at screens.

I remembered how in Mary Karr's book, *LIT*, she talks about how her sobriety group kept her sober. Interested in rereading *LIT*,

I posted a call for a book club on Facebook. More than twenty newly sober folks responded. To host this club, I created the Pandemic Sober Squad Facebook Group. Virtual sobriety was the way in these strange times, and if I were to stay sober, I needed this group. During a pandemic, especially, I wanted to hang out with folks that know what it's like to get sober on top of this very stressful, ongoing global pandemic.

I collected people during those early days from TLC sobriety meetings. I felt compelled to connect with those who needed help and those I was curious about. My friendly outreach starkly contrasted with my introverted ways. This was something I was compelled to do, flexing my internal need for connection outwardly.

Then there's the garden. Along with growing a community, I started growing a garden. I look back at pictures of dirt, raised beds, baby plants, seeds, and tools, and I remember how obsessed I was with doing this right. As with being super outgoing in organizing and running PSS, I was now a pseudo-farmer. But I felt compelled to do this, as well. Here's a snippet from my morning pages on March 22, 2020:

I bought all my garden stuff (for now) and also a spreader and a lawn mower. Who is this person? I don't like dirt. I don't like to be outside much, etc. I think I just want to be more self-sufficient. Who knows how long this plague will last? This is the most healthy way I can soothe ... I am going into the dirt to find myself.

I genuinely thought that civilization might come crashing down. Many of us did, but because my mind was so fuzzy in early sobriety, I just did the next best thing to take care of myself and didn't dwell on what I couldn't control. These next best things were cultivated over many prior trips into sobriety. I learned a lot through my relapses, and I'm no longer ashamed of them today. I treat them like little pets that have taught me a lot.

I look over my Instagram (@jbroyakima) day count and see those early garden pictures. One raised bed. Two raised beds. Three. Tomatoes, green peppers, carrots, broccoli, zucchini, Walla

Walla sweet onions, sweet peas, and spinach. Today, my whole backyard is a garden. I ripped out that grass and busted out of the raised beds. It's flourishing, like me.

The *New York Times* published a great Oliver Sacks essay on the power of gardens, and this part resonated with me: "I cannot say exactly how nature exerts its calming and organizing effects on our brains, but I have seen in my patients the restorative and healing powers of nature and gardens, even for those who are deeply disabled neurologically. In many cases, gardens and nature are more powerful than any medication."[1]

Like gardens, PSS is entering its fallow season as the pandemic wanes. It's transitioning to something new as everything changes again. And that is okay. Heraclitus is credited with saying, "There is nothing permanent except change." Caring for fellow humans and nature leads to taking care of myself. I will always seek to care, grow, and thrive.

I believe these life paths present themselves only beyond our comfort zones. Onward.

---

1. Oliver Sacks: The Healing Power of Gardens. New York Times https://www.nytimes.com/2019/04/18/opinion/sunday/oliver-sacks-gardens.html

MARY RAMENOFSKY

Recovering Irish-Catholic-Chicagoan planting new roots in San Diego. Sober mom, wife, daughter, sister, aunt, friend, and teacher. Solar-powered hiker, walker, yogi and meditator. Daily napper and reader (library book hoarder). Always up for attending sporting events and anything basketball related. Determined to show our next generation that life is better without alcohol.

As I reflect on the almost three years and three months since I had my last drink, I'm surprised to see how many things I have done on a regular basis to help keep me alcohol-free.

My early days of sobriety looked and felt quite different than what my days look like today, but whether I'm getting by minute-to-minute, day-to-day, or month-to-month, the things I do to remain sober have remained consistent and effective. I can't say I do all of these things every day, but I do them regularly and the positive impact they have on my sobriety is crystal clear.

Simply put I move my body, calm my mind, and connect my soul. My sobriety date fell just three days before WHO declared the COVID–19 pandemic, and only two days before my mom died from metastatic breast cancer. I had no idea that my world—

personally and globally—would come to a screeching halt, but I had committed a few weeks earlier to a three-month break from alcohol, effective 3/8/2020.

Overcome with grief and panic, I spent my first three weeks of sobriety sleeping. All night and all day. Finally, one day I crawled out of bed, stepped into my walking shoes, and took a walk around the block. I cried (sobbed, actually) the whole way around the block.

Day by day, I started to add another block, and before I knew it I was walking three to five miles every day. Walking around the neighborhood became my go-to tool for moving my body, calming my mind, and connecting my soul. The fresh air and pumping blood gave me the boost I needed to get through those skin-crawling days of early sobriety. I also used this time to binge podcasts like *On Being* and Brené Brown and to catch up on phone calls. I discovered that I opened up to friends and family much easier while on a walk than while sitting at home.

Three years have passed, and I continue to make the same loop around my neighborhood. I also started to read books during those early days while we were stuck at home. One of the books I picked up was called *Hiking My Feelings*. Instead of drinking to numb my feelings, I discovered the joy of hiking my feelings! My neighborhood walks eventually led to local hikes, regional hikes, and even thru-hikes!

I hiked the Trans-Catalina Trail and have made it a tradition to celebrate my annual sober milestones with special hikes. I quickly learned the best time to go hiking was early in the morning, which would never be possible if I were hungover. Hiking has also become my go-to activity for getting together with friends, old and new. I have yet to have anyone offer me a drink on the trail, which means I don't have any of those awkward moments when I need to decide how I will answer his or her questions on why I don't drink.

The frequency of my hiking has varied over the last few years, but just like walking, it's always there for me. As soon as I recognize I'm struggling with sobriety, anxiety, or just life being lifey, I lace up my boots and fill up my pack, and step-by-step I'm back on track.

One of the silver linings of the pandemic was the availability of online classes. Between the books I read (hellooooo quit lit!) and the podcasts I listened to, yoga was mentioned a lot. Yoga was one of those things that I had always dreamed of doing, but was too anxious and self-conscious to take a class. Well now that classes were offered online, I decided about a month into my sobriety journey to give it a go.

From day one I was hooked! I was doing one to three classes a day online and couldn't get enough. I even started to worry at one point that I had swapped my dependence on alcohol with a dependence on yoga. Fast-forward three years, and my yoga practice has calmed down, but the power it has to keep me moving, calm, and connected hasn't changed at all. Similar to celebrating my sober birthdays with a special hike, I now celebrate my "belly button birthdays" with an online yoga class with friends and family. It's the perfect alcohol-free celebration!

Besides the online yoga classes, I also discovered an online meditation class early on in my sobriety journey and pandemic life. Similar to yoga, I had always wanted to learn meditation but was too shy to join a class. Joining online was less intimidating, and just like yoga, I was hooked! Besides learning how to meditate, I found an incredible community. This meditation class was offered by a local Jewish synagogue.

I'm not Jewish, but I was following the person who leads the classes and learned of it through her newsletter. As the weeks went on and 2020 continued to throw curve balls at us, this group became quite close. I opened up to them about my sobriety and learned to trust them and love them, even though I had never actually met any of them in person.

I eventually did meet some of them in real life and joined their weekly hiking group. Not only did I discover the gift of meditation, but I found a community where I felt comfortable being myself. I continue to enjoy this weekly meditation group online, as well as use the breathing/grounding/visualization tools that I've learned from this class in my daily life.

Year One of sobriety was *filled* with movement and calming practices to keep me sober, but I knew deep down that something was still missing. I had made connections in my new yoga, meditation, and hiking communities, but I still felt that no one really understood what it was like to live a sober life, especially as our world was starting to come back together after a year into the pandemic. This is when I found The Luckiest Club, an online sobriety support community.

I'll never forget sitting in the back of our family's minivan at the drive-in theater, signing up for TLC on my phone while my kids watched *Trolls World Tour.* The tears rolled down my face as I scrolled through the app, reading threads of people talking about *all the things* that bounced around my head and my heart.

I attended my first online support meeting the next morning. I was scared, nervous, excited, curious, and felt a million other emotions. But I was no longer alone in sobriety.

For many months, I attended several meetings a day and joined every extra program they offered. Over two years later, I still attend at least four meetings a week. The love and support I receive and give in this community is beyond anything I can put into words. I have no doubt but that it keeps me sober.

Actually, there is one thing I continue to do, not just on a "regular basis," but also on a daily basis. Every single day since 3/8/2020, I have made the choice to stay sober and not drink alcohol. I may not always be consciously aware that I'm making that choice, but when I reflect on it I am incredibly grateful that I continue to make that choice every single day.

Living a sober life isn't always easy, but it is absolutely worth it.

Moving my body, calming my mind, and connecting my soul is what helps me continue to make that choice every day. For me, for my family, and for our future.

MELISSA WELLS

I am a 41-year-old fellow seeker who can feel and see all things clearly without living under the fog of alcohol. After 24 years of using alcohol to cope with life, I stopped "coping" and started "living" this one life I get, all with one simple, but not easy, decision: to never to drink poison again. With almost three years sober, I am a mama of four miraculous humans—two girls and two boys—passionate soccer player since age 10, long distance runner, nature lover, children's toy store manager, and have been in a relationship with my husband for 28 years. I am also a proud Leo, who will forever be grateful to lead a life in a state of recovery and healing.

My greatest personal achievement in sobriety calls to mind the words of Coach Taylor of the football drama, *Friday Night Lights*: "Clear eyes. Full hearts. Can't lose."

As the wife of a high school football coach, currently in our 17th football season together, I find great comfort in sports analogies and inspiration. As an athlete since age 8, I also believe that a huge part of my recovery and healing is in large part due to the fighting spirit, tenacity, and competitive drive that grew in me on a soccer field.

The clarity in my eyes and mind, gratitude and self-love in my heart and soul, and hopeful attitude for the present and future are all active parts of my daily life now. Before October 22, 2020, I felt very little clarity, gratitude, or hope.

Clear Eyes

Burning eyes, burning insides, foggy mind. From 2018–2020, the only time I faced myself in the mirror was when I was putting eye drops in my eyes. Those were the darkest two years of my addiction. When I hardly ever, if at all, drank for fun, for celebration, or for any purpose other than isolating, numbing, and self-medicating. I often didn't even use the mirror to put eye drops in, to do this near-daily task—not only because I was so well-practiced at landing eye drops in my eyes, but out of avoiding the person looking back at me in the mirror. This hopeless Band-Aid of a cover-up, used to successfully deceive all my co-workers, my kid's preschool teacher, and even myself: As long as my eyes *looked* clear, as long as the red blood vessels were gone, no one would see the burning. However, the pain, the constant, dull ache, the seemingly ever-present vision floaters, hangover headaches, and that agonizing shame—none of that could *ever* have been relieved with eye drops.

Now, in my alcohol-free life, I can stare in the mirror at the depths of my soul, directly at my own eyeballs, with pride, with wonder, in awe at the me I dug out from so far deep in that agony of addiction. Now I am staring at a warrior woman, mama, wife, daughter, sister, friend, and faithful, self-loving human. This feels like an achievement to me.

The clarity of mind I have untapped in sobriety has allowed me to kindly say, "No" as often as I need to, regardless of how much I may disappoint another human. I've been able to make career choices that align with my desire to truly enjoy how I spend my days. While working at a job I truly love, at an educational toy store, I can hear my intuition loud and clear. I can follow my soul's desire to help make people's days brighter, more fun, and more fulfilled through teaching and learning through play, and giving to others.

Full Heart

Self-disdain and self-sabotage blocked my heart from being able to nourish or practice self-love, let alone building a consistent connection and loving relationship with really anyone other than my children. Even my relationship with my children was not being lived out in a full heart kind of way. Without full presence or intentional time after 5 p.m. with any other human because of chasing that numbed-out, daily, drunk feeling, it became very difficult to be "full" of anything other than hot air. When a person is trapped in a daily cycle of addiction, it is common to be ruled by guilt and shame, especially when we start to fail at our own promises early in the morning. As a full-time working mom with a second shift of get-it-all-done for everyone else, I was driven by cheap red wine and vodka, and living on autopilot. This kept my heart feeling more than empty. Cold. Selfish. Incompetent. I covered every feeling of inadequacy and emptiness while pouring infinite booze into myself and pouring energy out of myself into caring for and worrying about others. But something alive in me was not ready to die—my ability to have a full heart.

When I stopped drinking completely and made it through the first 60 days of physical and mental exhaustion, I started to feel like I was getting to know an old friend again. I began to feel less temperamental, less frenetic, and less fragile. I was more patient, calmer, and endlessly more present.

Before my drinking became a full-blown addiction, my life vision was to have four children. As I write this, I am 30 weeks pregnant with my fourth child. It doesn't even feel right to say this is a personal achievement because it is not. It is an achievement of family, an achievement of contributing to our society and our humanity. I mother from a full heart and an intentional love so deep it knows no limits. But having the opportunity to grow this child inside of my sober and healthy body is absolutely an achievement I am proud of.

In 2014 and 2015 I experienced three miscarriages between my second and third children. I never stopped drinking to prepare myself to get pregnant with my third child. I only stopped drinking when I got a positive pregnancy test, and then up to the 10-week mark, at which time I repeatedly miscarried.

My body only knew the toxicity of near-daily drinking; it did not know how to provide a healthy womb and safe place in which to grow a baby past the first trimester. I know this now. I did not know this then.

I buried my repeated grief in more alcohol. I think of this time period in my life as similar to repeatedly opening a bad scab on your knee—the wound never getting a chance to fully heal; the injury starting over and over. You continue to take part in behavior risky enough to cut that knee scrab open again and again instead of stopping, resting, healing.

The scars kept getting deeper, the pain more numbed, and my heart more callused. As I prepare to mother a fourth child, and continue to do my best as mama to my other three children, I feel the small and big ways that leading with my full heart is teaching my children to grow and lead with love and compassion, too. This feels like an achievement to me.

Can't Lose

Guilt, torturous shame, stuck thoughts, and beyond hopelessness. I was stuck in a daily drinking tornado whose vortex trapped me. I felt like I was losing at everything. Losing my ability to enjoy life, to set goals and go after them, to make it one to two days without turning to alcohol to feel better, feel less, feel nothing. I was losing time—time with my kids and family that I couldn't get back. I chose distraction and numbing over real and meaningful conversations with my kids about the school day or new and old friends, brushing teeth, and bedtime stories.

I had convinced myself, or my addiction had convinced me,

that I wasn't capable of winning, overcoming, or changing. Guilt and shame led me to a darkness that knew no victory and a daily drinking habit that knew no other way.

On October 21, 2020, I simply had enough. I still had my daily three to eight drinks that day, but was repulsed by every sip, every losing thought, every dark corner of my heart, every possibility of bloodshot eyes and clouded thoughts upon waking the next morning.

With 750 days of sobriety today, I no longer have this losing mindset. Every day is a victorious day of life worth living. Not every day is easy or fun, but having the opportunity to feel every emotion, at every turn, with clarity and a full heart, now *that* is winning. All of this is the achievement I am most proud of today.

PAULA GELLA

Curious, lifelong seeker. Lover of change. Traveling occupational therapist with wanderlust in my veins. Mother of two daughters, one of whom is 24 and sober. Enneagram 7. Master procrastinator. Big fan of living alone but never lonely. Secretive, sneaky, lying drinker slamming bottles in bathrooms everywhere. Benefactor of so much grace.

Oh, the things I was so sure of before I removed alcohol from my life. Oh, the false assumptions I made! I was sure sobriety would make me a boring outcast who would never let loose, laugh, or have fun again at a gathering. I was so sure I couldn't manage my feelings.

How wrong those assumptions would turn out to be. How long those assumptions would keep me from getting sober and creating the life I wanted.

These are the things I want to tell that young naïve self— making all the false assumptions—and others making those same assumptions. You will have many closer authentic and supportive friends and relationships than you have ever had in your life. You will form a large and strong network with people from around the world—magnificent, brave, supportive, committed, hilarious, kind, and loving friends from all walks of life whom you will be in communication with through chats, online meetings and texts. Daily. You will feel more supported, understood and cared for than you have ever been before.

You will also play a key role in supporting others in saving their own lives. You will travel to meet people you have never met in person, and you will feel like you've already spent a lifetime with them and that you know them intimately—because you do. You've known them for a short time, a few years or less, and already know their deepest desires and fears and traumas and joys. And they know yours.

You will meet authors and mentors, heroines and heroes. You will find solace in books and podcasts and poetry. You will find inspiration from Pema, Glennon, Laura McKowen, Holly Whittaker, St. Brene, Amy D, David Whyte, Richard Rohr, Rich Roll, Nadia Bolz-Weber, and so very many more.

You will be exposed to all the components of "the work" of emotional sobriety that will enrich your life. You will attend retreats and large conventions and other gatherings that will bring you so much joy, and you will come away with new friendships and priceless knowledge.

You will have the confidence you've always sought through alcohol but didn't find. You will have the confidence to talk to anyone at any time in any situation. You will be able to go to bars and restaurants and concerts and celebrate holidays, weddings and other life events and still be able to let loose, laugh hard, make toasts, and remember these times without the blur of the alcohol haze.

Your mental health will improve so much that you will wish you would have known earlier that consuming alcohol is like pouring gasoline on your anxiety and depression. You will be able to feel all of your difficult feelings and have other ways to cope. You will know what it's like to throw everything you have in your arsenal and your soul at something, to try and fail so many times, but come out victorious.

You will see alcohol for what it really is, a glamorized toxin that slowly kills body, mind, and spirit. You will find a spirituality of your own because there will be so many synchronicities and signs that you are on the right path.

You will change the trajectory of your daughter's life by watching her get sober and live an authentic life she can call her own. Together you will break the cycle of addiction in your family and gain respect for your efforts. You will never know the lives that will be altered in future generations because you will be open, loud, and proud about your sobriety. You will feel no shame.

Your descendants may look back, if they are struggling, and say, "But look what they did. Just look. I have it in me too. They are with me."

You will finally find the freedom you didn't know was needed, or possible, or that is your birthright. You will carefully and sometimes painfully excavate your authentic self and learn to like her, maybe even love her.

S.D.

Mom, wife, ICU nurse. Heavy drinking was my favorite pastime. I always had my shit together and, without fail, looked like I was having fun. No one would have ever thought it was a problem.

The most powerful thing that helped me get and stay sober was connection. I've heard the quote, "The opposite of addiction is not sobriety; it's connection." I believe that with everything inside of me, with every fiber of my body. Initially the connections that were the most powerful were those formed with other people on the same journey. Something is so incredibly healing about staying connected with those who understand the battle. It's like we have this survivors' bond that is naturally formed when we break free of addiction. We know what it's like to be prisoners to a substance. We have fought the same monster. We celebrate the same victory. We share the same joy in living free.

Attending meetings is my lifeline. I found The Luckiest Club. Their meetings are all online, so I could take them with me wherever I went. Because I got sober in the pandemic, I had a lot of free time, and thankfully they held a lot of meetings throughout the day.

I needed to hear that I was not the only one, that other people were going through the same thing I kept hidden for so long. I don't know that I can fully express how healing it was to listen to other people talk about all the things that had been swarming around inside of me. I needed to hear from people who were further along on the journey than I was. I needed to know that lasting change was possible. I needed to hear someone validate how hard this was and that *it was still worth it.* I needed to hear people who were back on Day One share about how bad it feels, that picking up the bottle again wasn't worth it. I needed to hear people in early sobriety share the joy and excitement over all of the first sober wins.

Though I'm not really tempted to drink anymore, I still attend meetings. It's like exercising and fitness—we have to keep doing the things that got us to what we were trying to achieve. The best analogy I heard is *what if I worked out at the gym and ate healthy meals every day and met my fitness goals, what would happen if I suddenly stopped all the behaviors that got me to that goal? I'd lose the muscle over time; I'd lose that new physique I worked for. If I want to keep that in-shape body, I need to keep going to the gym and eating right.* The same concept applies to meetings, connection, and maintaining sobriety.

Showing up to the world raw, clear, and present is really f***ing hard, especially in the first few months of getting sober. I faced feelings that I didn't even know I had. I felt sadness, irritability, rejection, disappointment, anger, insecurity, and rage. I spent my adult life drowning these feeling in a bottle of wine. I had no idea what to do with them.

I also felt joy, *real joy,* something I don't think I ever felt in my 36 years of life. In sobriety I've learned what it is to feel excited, happy, playful, curious, delighted, peaceful, and relaxed. I've gotten to laugh! And, *oh my gosh,* laughing at something when we're sober is 1,000 times better than laughing at something when we're drunk.

Feelings, especially the uncomfortable or unpleasant ones, are scary. I spent my whole life running from them. Connecting with others in sobriety makes it less scary. So I check in with my sober girlfriends, or I log into a meeting on zoom. Some days I just listen to shares and other days I pour out all of my feelings and put them in a safe place. I call it dumping, like I have to dump my emotional garbage; I have to get out the toxic stuff. I learned that keeping this stuff bottled up inside is what causes me to self-destruct. I don't need my girlfriends or the community to give me answers or advice; I just need someone to give me a place to lay this stuff down.

Drinking (and recovering from drinking) took up so much time. When I was finally able to put the bottle down, I was blown away by how much free time I had each day. It's like drinking had taken over every corner of my life and I was left with no hobbies. I had to learn to fill that time with other things that bring me joy, happiness, comfort, and peace.

In getting sober, I was free to explore and rediscover myself and the things that I like. I could dabble into different outlets and discover what I enjoy. I learned that I love tinkering on projects around my home. I love making arts and crafts with my kids. I dive into the spirit of every season with my seven-year-old; I am free to play and create with him. Life is so much more fun now that I am truly present in these moments and can remember them.

I spend time outside in the fresh air. I learned that I love working in my yard. I remember when I was drinking, I couldn't even keep a houseplant alive. But along the way, with so much free time and with all the exploring, I found that digging in the dirt and trimming my tropical plants gives me so much joy. I now look around my yard, and though I live in California, my plants are thriving, and they could rival the appearance of any lush tropical garden in Kauai. It's amazing the things we can do when our hands are free to move and play rather than being glued to a glass.

I started to exercise again. And I liked it. I remember for years while I was drinking, my running really started to suffer. As the hangovers got worse, the running became more difficult, and by my last two years of drinking, I wasn't able to run at all. My liver and pancreas hurt all the time. I lived with a constant low-grade fever.

As my body started to heal from no longer filling it with poison, the constant stinging and aching pains started to ease. And by 10 months into sobriety, I started running again. The running became fun. It was something I enjoyed. I felt free. I was finally able to start meeting the athletic goals that I had set for myself so long ago. After I stopped drinking, I could run farther, faster, and harder than I had ever imagined. I can sprint uphill, I can conquer intimidating inclines, and I have surpassed every fitness goal that I set for myself back when I was drinking. I have found that running is a great outlet, and it helps with my mental health and my moods.

Now that the daily "well-deserved wine glass" is gone, I had to find other treats to fill that void. When I was drinking, I never ate desserts and boasted being "low carb." Though I knew better, I think I kept a high level of denial that all the wine, beer, and booze are really just ethanol that breaks down to sugar when it's processed in the body. Once it was removed, I had gnarly sugar cravings.

So in sobriety I let myself indulge in sugary treats, fancy coffees, and all the seltzer waters. I stocked up on my favorite flavors of water, and I keep them in a special private stash. I am saving at least $500 a month on alcohol, so I splurge elsewhere. Lollipops became a regular habit in early sobriety; they gave me a sugar fix and kept my hands busy.

I developed little routines that keep me grounded daily. I wake early in the mornings and enjoy coffee time alone and in the quiet. I pray, I meditate; I set an intention for the day. I savor these hang-over-free mornings. They are a gift that never gets old! I reflect on life, my thoughts, and my feelings. I keep a journal, and I have a gratitude practice. I learned that implementing a small daily grati-tude list can improve overall psychological wellbeing and mental health. I was once a prisoner to alcohol; I don't want to forget where I came from. I don't want to stop celebrating this newfound freedom.

I've heard a lot of people talk about what they do daily that keeps them sober. I have learned that there isn't a right or wrong way to do this or some manual of "have-tos." *It's about living.* All these little things that I brought into my life when alcohol got removed are just life's activities. And that's what sobriety, its freedom to really live.

WHITNEY BISHOP

50-something wife, mom, nana, consultant, and reluctant caregiver. Curious. Creative. Courageous.

"Bringing Home Dad"

In late 2019, I was asked to reengage in a family dynamic I had successfully extricated myself from decades earlier. Dad was in poor health, making poor choices, and living in filth. My mom (his former wife) and my brother invited me back in to see if I could talk any sense into him. It was one of the few times in decades that the four of us were in a room together.

I reluctantly accepted their invitation to reengage, and then my drinking ramped up steadily. By the time the pandemic hit in March 2020, I was going through a big box of wine every couple of days. My relationship with alcohol was as complicated as my relationship with my father.

The emotional pain, physical stress, anger and frustration were constant. I believed that alcohol was the only thing that could help me manage these emotions. The truth was that alcohol wasn't providing any relief—just more misery. I would later hear something that would connect me back to this truth: "You can't get enough of something that *almost* works."

When the pandemic fears peaked, my delusional and agitated dad was moved in the middle of the night from the hospital to the rehab facility. The next day, all visitation was shut down, and we had no way to see him. We could talk with him by phone, but he was so confused that it was difficult for him to understand why we weren't there and why we isolated him in that facility.

On May 8, 2020, I woke up fully clothed on top of the bed, my head pounding, an empty glass in hand, and my screwdriver spilled all over the bedspread and floor. In that moment, I knew that this was not who I needed to be or how I needed to show up if I was going to be of service to my family and myself.

That day, I became more involved as Dad's advocate, rather than a dutiful, disinterested daughter. I enlisted the help of my mom and brother, rather than thinking I needed to do it all myself. And when the facility repeatedly told me that I couldn't see or touch Dad, despite his obvious and rapid decline, I did the only thing I could think of: I asked if they were hiring.

I begged God, "If this is meant to be, let it be easy."

And it was. They hired me on the spot and walked me right back to his room. Seeing him and touching him for the first time in five months was overwhelming and confusing for us both. I'll never forget the incredulous look on his face or his tone as he asked, "Whitney, is that you? What are you doing here?"

"I just got a job here, Dad."

"What? You have a business. You have a degree. You can't have a job here. You don't want to work here."

The hiring manager stood at the foot of Dad's bed by me. I replied, "I'll bet you worked a few jobs you didn't want to while raising us, yeah?"

He smirked, laughed a little pained laugh, and nodded his head.

"Well, it's my turn."

By the time I had worked five work shifts, I witnessed enough to decide that he needed to leave there if he was going to live his remaining days with any dignity or joy.

On a break one night, I asked him what he really wanted. "I just want to go home—whatever that means," he replied.

In that moment, I knew what I had to do. My next move was to pick up the phone and ask my husband if it was ok for us to move him in. I am grateful to say that the answer was an unequivocal "yes" from everyone who would surround us with love, support, encouragement, and nourishment for the next 47 days, when he would transition from this life.

So many conflicting feelings and emotions.

So much work to do.

Cleaning out his place.

Working at the nursing home.

Bringing him home.

Managing his daily needs.

Navigating family relationships.

Handling his affairs and all he left behind.

That wiser, more evolved part of me knew that eliminating alcohol would give me greater access to my inner wisdom and would reduce the chatter and noise of the inner critic. It would be a gift for me and for all those I love and serve.

Because I was sober, I could do all of this with

a clear head

a clear heart

and

no regrets.

My sobriety and recovery helped to elevate the quality of my conversations and my questions, each in greater alignment with my values and soul's purpose.

My questions shifted from:

"Why the hell do I feel like I'm the one who should take care of him?"

"Why is everyone standing around with their heads up their butts?"

to:

"How can I show up for him, our family, during this really difficult time?"

"Who do I need on the team?"

"What support can I expect, request?"

"What is my heart asking of me?"

"What would I want someone to do for me in this situation?"

On the morning he passed, I was in the other room, journaling. I remember being tuned into a change in the energy, the temperature of the room. I remember feeling a sense of dread, followed by a sense of peace. I said my last goodbye as the team came to do their work.

The resentment and anger we harbored with each other had been transformed into something different during our time together. We both surrendered. We did the bravest and hardest thing we could do: We allowed ourselves to love one another, unconditionally. We allowed ourselves the gift of making living amends to one another. We walked away from the experience forever changed.

Clear-headed.

Clear-hearted.

No regrets.

B.N.

I am a single mom to 10- and 7-year-old girls and have been sober since March 8, 2018.

I wrote this in July 2020, four months into the COVID-19 Pandemic. I was two years and two months sober and seriously considering what sobriety, and even life, meant during those uncertain times. Reflecting on my thoughts during this time brings me back to the basics of sobriety, joy, and life.

The goal line has shifted these days for most of us. In these last four months, almost all of our familiar measures of success have been thrown out of the window, and we see ourselves struggling to even answer the basic question: How are you doing?

Normally, we answer this question based on a series of known variables: We accomplished some magic number of things at work, or we didn't. We saw one of our children achieve something they had been working towards, or we watched them learn the lesson of defeat. Maybe we just booked an exciting vacation or are just returning from one that failed to meet our expectations. Maybe our finances are looking solid, and we are planning for that new kitchen renovation, or they aren't, and we are stuck with our laminate floors. Our job is going great, or it is not. We have a hot date coming up or are fantasizing about one we should not be fantasizing about.

Goal lines, metrics, and measures of success—these things shift. It happens to all of us. With age, maturity, changes in life situations, and external circumstances, we start looking at life a little differently and continue to edit and evolve our metrics and our goals.

Now, however, with the global pandemic stretching into the fourth month, the metrics haven't just shifted. They have all been erased. What *is* a good day, anyway? A strong Internet connection and a good set of earbuds?

Compared to what we are used to, the bar for an okay day seems pretty low. A good day might be one in which no one we know is sick, has died, or has gotten hurt. We are employed today. Our business has not shut its doors. Our kids let us work for 30-minute spans instead of 10. The grocery store is no longer out of hand soap and sanitizer.

All around me, I am beginning to hear people evaluate their lives a little differently. Some people are, for the first time, thinking about what is really important to them. For me, this all feels very familiar. It reminds me of when I first got sober!

When I first got sober, old metrics that I depended on, and thought were important had to die if I wanted to save my life. I had to become comfortable with simple successes: a day without drinking—success! I did not yell at my children today—success! Only ate one bag of gummy worms—success!

Now, I am not only dealing with a pandemic, but I am also dealing with the first stages of an upcoming divorce. With this divorce, almost every single metric of success I built for myself has to be thrown out the window. Luckily, most of these "metrics" were embarrassingly materialistic or convenience based and needed to go. But some good stuff was in there too! I very quickly realized that I had built a whole identity on things and people external to myself. And it was meaningless.

The reason I realized this very quickly and not slowly is because when you wake up and realize you don't even know *who you are,* or how to show up in the world, there is nowhere to hide. I had to address this head on, or I knew I would suffer.

I am going to tell you what I did to move past meaningless metrics of success and move into thinking about sobriety and myself differently.

I literally took out a piece of paper and wrote a list titled: Who I Am and What I Want. *I am a married woman. We live in X neighborhood. I want stability. I want a forever marriage like I was promised. I want my kids to grow up in a regular home with both parents. I want to upgrade my car when it dies. I don't want to move to a smaller house. I want to be someone who is able to quit my job if I want to.* Then, I physically crossed of everything that was not true anymore.

Then, I rewrote the list and filled it with things I *know* about *myself.* Things that cannot be taken away by anyone or any situation. The list was long. The list made me proud. The list still had some asshole stuff on it. But the list also included: *I am a woman who is proudly sober. I am a good mother. My team respects me. I know and love hard work. I do things for my family.*

I did the same thing with What I Want. These became my new metrics of success: *Did I feel joy today? Did I love, like really feel love with my kids today? Did I act out old patterns, and if so, did I catch myself?*

This was an important one: *Did I accomplish what I set out to do today?* Not what someone else would have me do. What *I,* alone, set out to do? And related to this: *Did I feel spiritually connected enough to even know what I needed to accomplish today?*

And of course: *Was I sober today?*

Here's what I believe is true: When metrics get thrown away, better things that are truer and actually mean something take their place. For me, it was things like I mentioned above. I am not clear on my list yet. Not even close. This will be the great work of my life, and I'll never be done.

But—I have started. I revisit my list often, sometimes daily if I need to. I tweak, and I see what feels right that day. I see patterns that keep coming up, usually related to fitting in or comparing. Through that process, I learn about myself.

This is something I wish for all of us. I wish we could look at our old list of metrics and realize that much of it was crap and needed to go anyway. I wish we could see what we have left, and realize the list is different, but it's long, and it should make us proud. Because our current list may include how much hand sanitizer was readily available at the store, and did I remember to buy a new mask, but it also includes things like: Did we finally dig our old bikes out of the garage today? Did we plant vegetables for the first time? Did we finally have that picnic in that field we drive by every day? Did we find new ways of connection that will outlast this season? Did we witness a collective suffering and also a collective set of real actions that will outlive every single one of us? Did someone we thought would never change his or her mind say, "I was wrong, I understand now, and I'm working alongside you?"

Some days none of this makes any sense at all, and I don't find exercises like this particularly useful. Some days, the thought of a divorce, especially right now when we don't even know what tomorrow is going to look like, feels overwhelming, crushingly lonely, and very unfair. Even the sobriety thing feels like, "Okay, fine. I'm not going to drink. But I'm going to be grumpy about it."

Those are the days when I am most grateful for the earliest lesson I learned in sobriety, which now extends to every part of my life. "It's just today. I just have to make it through today. Just do the next right thing today."

This serves me well, every single day.

PROFESSOR CHEF
RICK WARNER

I teach History at a small, liberal arts college for men, and integrated cooking with my classes and writing projects. Before starting my career as a professor, I worked as a professional chef for 12 years. I participate in at least five sober platforms though TLC, which is my main jam now. Sobriety freedom date: 27 July 2019.

A key concept especially in early sobriety is not to "future trip," but to take our struggle one day at a time. The common refrain is that I cannot focus on tomorrow, I just need to get my head on the sober pillow at the end of the day. Or perhaps earlier on, it is one hour at a time.

After about a year, I found my fleeting thoughts about picking up a drink had all but left me. I can now spend time in pubs and with inebriated people in social settings, and the worst I can say is that they get boring to me—and perhaps remind me about why I quit.

After about a year, I was surprised to see that although cravings and occasional visits from that "moderation trickster" had died down, I still had more work to do.

I had noticed in recovery meetings from the beginning that

people with significant sobriety still attended and participated. They rarely discussed cravings or even alcohol, for that matter, unless they were remembering dark days. I was never sure if they did that to help others know that recovery is possible or if they were still stuck in the past somehow with their bitterness. Likely a bit of both.

This new phase that some call "emotional sobriety" truly does have an emotive edge. My program of recovery had encouraged me to investigate my feelings about the past and make changes based on those reflections. I think something in the natural order of things encourages us to search our feelings more when we are generally rid of the temptation to drink. I think we have a tendency to adopt a more philosophical approach, and after a while, I think we naturally are driven to give back to a world that we once were oblivious to.

Having spent considerable time in introspection, I began to turn to how I viewed my new life. What indeed will I do in the future? I am nearing retirement age, and have reflected on how I will spend my last 25 years on this earth. Sobriety has brought me such peace! This peace allows me to reflect more honestly. Life is still lifey, as I often say. But I am approaching my challenges with a peace I did not know before.

In retirement I want to have fun. Is anything wrong with that? No. But as part two, I want to act meaningfully. I want to be of service to others, not for any particular gain financially or for popularity—honest! I want to give back.

I want to establish pathways of service work in the local and global communities. I may want to join the Peace Corps, for example. I would like to work with the local Latino community wherever I live, since my wife and I are both bilingual and some-what bicultural.

I would like to stay connected to a college community to participate in cultural and educational opportunities. I would likely continue to cook for others, hosting dinners and supporting organizations. For example, I roast about 20 turkeys each year for a free Thanksgiving dinner put on by several churches. I make a lot of ice cream and give it away. These are things that I can continue in sobriety, and do well in.

Along with these service ideas, I have become more interested in giving back to the sober community. In AA, this is the 12th step, but I would be doing it whether I read that or not. Those who know me recognize that I am very involved in multiple recovery communities. I like to approach this as just another person, or as we would say in TLC, just another noodle.

We are a circle of noodles, a healthy noodle soup. If I help you, that is helping me. The connection is important, no matter how many days of sobriety we claim. Some programs do have a long tradition of "sponsorship." In recent years, other programs have initiated informal sponsorship or "accountability partners."

The "rules" for these engagements are shifting. In this period of sobriety, we are expanding the concept of sponsorship in new and creative ways. It will be interesting to see where this leads. I do maintain individual contact with numerous people on the sober train, most of whom are in early days. I have seen this work. Connection does indeed defeat addiction.

This leads me to the final major outcome that I envision. I am an academic, a historian by trade. I am fascinated with the history of sobriety. A major historic change occurred in 1938 with the beginnings of Alcoholic Anonymous. There were community efforts at sobriety before that time, though generally few and (so far) hidden from history.

In the past, generational multiple alternatives to AA have arisen. I have participated in a number of these. As is said in The Luckiest Club, I respect all paths to recovery. The world is hard enough on us that we do not need to criticize one another needlessly.

I have found value in all of the platforms and programs that I have participated in. The connections I have made in my sober tribes have helped me achieve sobriety for 39 months now. I have turned to discussing sobriety with people in many places to open up these questions. I have given public addresses at my college and in a local church. Nearly everyone knows I am recovering. I do receive a lot of encouragement from the "normie" community as well.

Over the next few years, I intend to use my skills as a historian to help us learn about the many different attempts at sobriety that have been launched in different places through time. Much of this research will, by nature, be difficult since such information has always been kept from public eyes. The shame of addiction has a long history. My goal is to unearth whatever we can about efforts at sobriety since the time of the Greeks and across the world. What sorts of attempts or "programs" have been used? How has this issue been seated in the larger cultural history of individual societies? Most importantly, what lessons can we learn from other places and people that might help us in our sobering world? What can we learn from history?

I suspect that only history nerds can fully appreciate the challenge of such a project. But I do intend to do this work in the next segment of my life, one day at a time.

DUSTY SWEHLA

Mom, warrior, yogi, friend, Native American, addict. Thrill seeker, up for anything at least once, life-long learner. Healing, strong—except when I'm weak. A genius at making you believe whatever I want. (One of the many reasons no one knew about my addiction.)

Even before I stopped drinking, I thought about this question often. For years, honestly.

Without a drink, how will I work through all of life and the lifey challenges that will come my way?

With my many failed attempts at sobriety, *life* made me think I needed the drink. *Feeling* made me want to drink—not just the negative feelings that came with work, life, shitty weather, and relationships. The positive feelings made me want to drink, as well. Holidays, sporting events, celebrations, and a beautiful sunny day. I lived as a functioning alcoholic for many years. Working a full-time job, raising my kids, putting on a show of "normalcy." No one really knew the extent of my drinking—or did they?

. . .

As I lounged in bed the morning after what was my last night drinking, I thought about this question: "How will I live without alcohol?"

I had a difficult conversation with my husband that morning, and it was time to do something different, something I had never done. After my family left for the day, I prayed, asking, "What do I do? I'm so sick of feeling like this!"

So, I rolled out of bed, got on my knees, and asked Jesus for help. I couldn't do this alone anymore. What I was doing was not working. I had to surrender! That next day, I checked into outpatient rehab where I gained knowledge about my disease, listened as if it was a life sentence to everything that was said to me, and I did the work.

In the beginning, the biggest challenge was getting through a day. My daily routine had to change. I no longer drove the same way home from work. I shopped at different grocery stores, and for quite a while, I stayed away from "drinking" events.

I had to minimize the thought of drinking. The phrase, "One day at a time" was great, but a day was too long. So, my thoughts had to shift to, no drinking for … one hour at a time, one minute at a time, and sometimes one second at a time. I also told myself in the beginning, "I don't have to quit forever; just for today."

These little internal conversations got me through each day, sober.

Since I stopped drinking in September 2014, I have had many ups and downs and ebbs and flows that have tested my strength and sobriety. The first year of sobriety, I held on for dear life, counting every day, keeping gratitude at the front of my mind at all times.

I leaned into my yoga and meditation practice, attending many AA meetings, and visiting my therapist often. Year Two, things started to change. I noticed differences in the people around me, thinking, "Wow, she's really changed" or "Has she always acted like that?"

All of my relationships changed. The relationship with my co-workers, husband, and family. Everyone was different, so I thought. Turns out, many of them were the same; I was the one who had changed. I was seeing life through a different pair of glasses. I had some clarity for the first time in many years.

After following my inner compass, to do something different, I went back to school, changed careers, and started my own business. This was all very challenging, but I knew as long as I was sober, anything was possible. As many of us in recovery try to "do all the things," that is exactly what I did. I kept myself busy, so I didn't have to really *feel.* I loved what I was doing, but I felt tired and like I was running on a hamster wheel trying to keep up.

Once again, I needed a change.

In 2022, I had a bit of an awakening experience. This came with a once-in-a-lifetime opportunity. My boys are grown men, I'm in my mid-40s, I don't have grandkids yet. I thought, *If I don't do this now, I will never get the chance to do it again.*

What if I sell everything I own—my business, my closets full of things—and move to Costa Rica? Not necessarily thinking about my sobriety, I figured "I've got this."

A few short months after making my decision, I was living in Costa Rica.

This has been by far the most challenging life event since I started this journey of sobriety. Being alone with your feelings in the middle of the jungle makes you do some deep soul searching. It's not that I have thought of needing a drink; I have wanted to escape the feelings and emotions that have come through this process. When everything around you is extremely quiet, you can hear so much.

I've come to terms with knowing that the only way through something is going through it. I'm working on many of the feelings I've suppressed for most of my life. I'm working through many of my fears and emotions that led me to the bottle in the first place. This move has been very simple, not at all easy.

I'm grateful that I have a large wellness toolbox, AA meetings I attend regularly, a supportive family, and Jesus—just as I did on Day One.

As I write this, I'm listening to the howler monkeys, a toucan is watching me from the tree outside my apartment, and I am sober. My foundation is strong, and I remind myself often: My best day drinking was worse than my worst day sober.

I'm learning once again to *feel*. It's quite liberating.

My life is truly beautiful, and without my sobriety, none of this would be possible. I'm grateful for this journey and the strength to work through all the waves that will continue to come my way.

As for now I'm going to continue on this journey, one day, one hour, one minute, and one second at a time.

JULI OTT

Mama, wife, sister, daughter, friend. Always seeking, always curious. Happily, retired party girl, yet still the life of the party. Aries. Enneagram 4. Always up for coffee—coffee is life. My two best adult decisions—sobriety and my pandemic puppy— have given me the most beautiful moments of truly being present.

Hi. I'm Juli, and I'm an alcoholic.

It's a sentence I have no shame in saying, and trust me, shame is a thing for me.

It's a sentence my daughter has heard and parroted back, often out of nowhere. It makes sense; I stopped drinking days after her sixth birthday, and it was the summer of online recovery meetings.

It's a sentence that gave me the opportunity to begin again.

It's a sentence that got me ready for what came next.

What came next is nothing that any person in recovery won't deal with—life. But this was life in a very raw state. This was finally dealing with so much I wasn't addressing. This was finally learning who I actually was. And I was doing this in a pandemic, while raising two children, and in a less-than-solid marriage.

Suffice it to say I was a bit of a mess.

Part of the mess was my ability to future trip. To catastrophize. Spending countless hours waiting for the moment that would test my resolve or expecting how my life was bound to blow up.

Anticipating disappointment when I ultimately failed.

Assuming my children are resigned to the same fate because I could see the similarities in how they spoke about themselves and moved throughout their little worlds. Yes, this gutted me at times.

It wasn't an easy headspace to operate in, and I certainly wasn't very kind to myself. Being kind to myself is still a struggle sometimes, even three years later. And of course, I have tools for this, and they work (who would have thought?). I have learned, though, that the right headspace doesn't just help me; it helps everyone around me.

Everyone in recovery will tell you it's something you have to do for you—and that's true. They will also tell you that doing it for you will improve your relationships—which is also true, though quick fixes for that to come to fruition aren't guaranteed (sorry to report that bit of bad news). The super honest folks in recovery will tell you that it will be painful, that it will be beautiful, that it will be hard, but that you will survive it all, as long as you keep the drink down. True, true, true, and true.

Yes, I have done it for me, and I have moved throughout my life in a different way because of it. Whereas three years ago, I felt like a shell of my former self, today I feel like a shell of the woman who entered an online recovery meeting, who eventually took her (hopefully last) Day One on June 14, 2020. I have more compassion for that woman, but I don't inhabit that same soul these days.

And my children have a different mother.

Their mother is now growing into the woman she was always meant to be. She is certainly more honest. She appears lighter and brighter and laughs authentically. She is healing more each day. She is accountable and apologizes when necessary (even to herself). She works hard on emotional regulation and is grateful she learned that phrase because, seriously, what a game changer!

Their mother was able to receive her children's ADHD diagnoses in a way that surprised her—because previously it would have pummeled her. She can respond instead of react and support them in a way alcohol wouldn't have allowed.

Their mother now sees that so many unanswered things about her, things she felt broken for, might have an explanation. She is the right person to learn new lessons and model for her children how to reframe these imperfections into celebrations of the people they are.

Their mother is the right person to get down on the floor with them when the world feels heavy and can usually say the right things (let's face it, we don't always get it right) because her mind is clear, and her heart is light.

Removing alcohol from my life got me ready for all of this. I no longer had a substance stealing my one precious life. My children and husband no longer had to compete for attention, because of a substance I centered our lives on. As my children grow and face situations involving alcohol, I have solid legs to stand on, to help them understand, truly, the potential consequences. One thing changed everything.

And it all started with one sentence.

LINDY PHELPS

Lindy has been happily married to her husband, Rob, for 19 years. She is mom to five amazing children—three girls and two boys—ranging from six years old to eighteen years old. By day she is an elementary educator, and by night, she is a passionate reader and writer.

Many people can occasionally drink alcohol for fun. Some people have a healthy relationship with alcohol. I am not one of those people. For way too long, it became a crutch for my anxiety and lack of self-worth. I wasn't a "drink all day, can't function without it" type of girl, but I was a "watch the clock until it's an acceptable time to drink" and "doesn't know when to call it a night" kind of girl. I wasn't drinking alcohol light-heartedly or for fun, I was drinking it to escape my crippling anxiety. News flash: I didn't.

I was pretty good at hiding my troublesome relationship with alcohol because it was mostly in the comfort of my own home in the evenings. This unhealthy relationship with alcohol never came to what society would define as a rock bottom, but I was not living a genuinely authentic life.

I think my family would agree I am a much happier and more present Lindy, now that I am alcohol-free. And while people may see the outward signs of my health journey, the inner work—my healed soul—is what has been life-changing and miraculous. There is absolutely no way that I could have achieved my sobriety on my own. It is truly only by the grace of God. He doesn't make mistakes, and I know He will use this journey of mine for the greater good.

Removing alcohol from the equation of my life did not miraculously make my anxiety go away; in fact, it made it worse for some time. I think it's supposed to be that way, because it was in those painful, raw, desperate moments that I decided I couldn't do it alone.

I started to pick up any quit lit I could find. In doing so, I discovered Laura McKowen's_*We Are The Luckiest,* which then led me to her online sober community called The Luckiest Club. This was the biggest game changer in my sobriety. This opened doors to healing, friendships, support, and emotional growth and well-being. In these online rooms, I was able to fill my sobriety toolbox with methods and practices to turn my life around and live authentically and unapologetically as my true self.

Early in my sobriety, I felt as though I had to rediscover who I really was. For so long, I used alcohol to define me. I used it naively, thinking it made me more fun, carefree, and social. It was my tool to take the easy way out because I avoided conflict my whole life.

When challenges arose, I immediately turned to a beverage to "cope." In doing so, I underestimated myself and deprived myself of the ability to learn how to navigate real life. I was slapping a Band Aid on a gaping wound, when I really needed to peel back the layers and heal from the inside out. I needed to learn that I was capable of putting one foot in front of the other to press on, even in my most stressful moments.

I had used alcohol to get me through an eating disorder, a broken engagement, my children's illnesses, the death of loved ones, my crippling anxiety and depression, and the day-to-day stresses. When I removed alcohol from the equation, I realized that the very thing I was using to "help" was actually the major contributing factor in my inability to face my problems head on and work through them in a healthy and healing way.

In the first couple months of living an alcohol-free life, I battled greatly with self-worth. I felt so broken and raw. Every emotion was magnified and, at times, felt unbearable. While my natural tendency had always been to hide from those tough thoughts and feelings, I quickly learned that I had to sit with them, become familiar with them, and figure out what my heart needed to get through them to a place of healing. And as life often does, it gave me plenty of opportunities to practice.

About six months into my sobriety, I found out that my dad, who has always been an athletic, driven, go-getter, was diagnosed with Parkinson's disease. The day I found out I couldn't peel myself off the couch. I went back and forth between crying and sleeping to try to forget. For many days I couldn't talk about it without crying.

But I did talk about it. I let it all out. I couldn't let that fear and sadness camp out in my heart and fester because that is what would have led me to drink in the past. And although it was one of the hardest things I've faced as an adult, it was a pivotal moment in my sobriety. I worked through the initial shock and sadness by leaning on those around me and getting the support I needed. It was the first time in sobriety that it never even crossed my mind to pour a drink to help me cope.

Slowly but surely, putting one foot in front of the other, I used coping mechanisms I had learned in sobriety support meetings to work through the anxiety and sadness. It has been a year and a half since his diagnosis, and he is doing really well. And I am so grateful that I am clear-headed and able to be a support system for him and my mom.

Fast forward to 14 months into my sobriety when I attended my first big party. At this point, I was not just surviving, but thriving in my alcohol-free lifestyle. I was looking forward to the chance to go out and have fun. It had been a while because of COVID–19, so we were long overdue for a night out!

I was not expecting it to be a struggle at all, which is why it hit me like a ton of bricks when I was overcome with sadness. Surrounded by so many wonderful friends and so much alcohol, I felt the grief of not being able to drink and feel carefree with them. I suddenly felt socially awkward and like I couldn't hold an engaging conversation. I immediately went to a place of zero self-confidence and feeling like I didn't belong.

Saying this now feels ridiculous, because I know that if any of my friends had known I was feeling that way, they would have gone out of their way to help me feel better. But I didn't want to be that burden for them. My husband and I left a little early, and rather than hold all those thoughts in, I opened the floodgates and poured it all out to him. And then I opened up a little more and shared it with some of my friends afterward.

Once again, I put one foot in front of the other and healed the broken pieces. I sat with those yucky feelings, acknowledged them, and connected with my support system to help move past the hurt. It was a humbling reminder that I need to stay diligent in my self-care practices and not become lazy in my sobriety journey.

I celebrated two years of sobriety on September 28, 2022. Writing is my passion, so it only seems fitting that God would use my mess and turn it into a hopeful message. For that, I am so very thankful. One day at a time, putting one foot in front of the other. Moving forward—not looking back.

SHANE WILLBANKS

Sober dad, truth-seeker, friend.

I finally got sober after decades of hard, destructive, drinking. I was going to die, plain and simple, and my life was a wasteland of failures and half-assed attempts to justify my misery.

At first, I had to get to six weeks without drinking in order to get a proper assessment of my liver enzymes. I made it. No community, no sober friends, no quit lit, no podcasts—just me, doing it. I made it 50 days, had my blood work, ultrasound, and whatever other tests they needed done.

My liver enzyme levels had improved. At one point, they'd had been so high that the physicians ran other tests to confirm them. So, I decided to go until New Year's Day, around four months in, just to say I did. Then, I decided to go for six months, then nine months, and so on.

At some point in my third month, I joined a sober community called TLC and discovered a world of others who understood. At some point in those first six months, I knew this was the life I wanted to live, the way I wanted to feel, and the way I wanted to be. My relationships either began to fall away because they were no longer beneficial, or they began to heal because I could hear, feel, and respond to what others needed.

I'm at a point in my life where I am no longer satisfied with my job or my station. I discovered powers I had hidden with alcohol and a passion for others trying to do the same. Powers like compassion for myself and grace for others and the pain they deal with, sitting with feelings rather than reacting to them or drinking at them.

At around five months of sobriety, I applied for an addiction studies program to become a substance abuse counselor. I did it to have an extra level of accountability, but I also did it because I love this path, I love that I achieved what seemed impossible before, and I love being able to answer the question, "How did *you* do it?"

In my old life, I was the best of liars, the best of manipulators, and the best of justifiers. I could talk myself into or out of anything, regardless of the harm it would bring or the disappointment that came. But something clicked somewhere in this journey—something settled on me like a warm blanket and changed my life. I found that I don't need to reinvent myself; I just need to focus my strengths and skills that I already possess onto those things that bring me healing, joy, and peace.

I found myself defending my sobriety and all of its gifts—as I once defended my drinking and all of its carnage. I discovered that I had the desire to not just live, or remain alive long enough to hold my grandchildren, but I had the desire to experience life, from the mundane to the extraordinary—from the painful to the miraculous, and all that is in between.

I discovered that the trials and struggles and pain gave me strength and perspective. They gave me the appreciation for a peaceful moment alone with myself or the love and beauty of a hug from a loved one. For the first time in a long time, I wanted to give what I had so freely been given: compassion, understanding, a helping hand, a smile and soft voice in a time when the world swirls around me like a Van Gogh brushstroke.

I guess I look forward to continuing to understand who I am and why I'm here, but I want to do so in the company of others who are doing the same, while helping those who want to realize that capacity exists in them. I look forward to continuing to tell the truth in all things, because I've discovered that the hardest consequences of doing that are easier to navigate than the smallest ones caused by deceit.

I have a lot of regrets—mostly brought on by my own actions or inactions—but I'm learning to live for the now while picking through the blast sites and wakes of destruction for clues to how to move forward. I visit those sites as I want to or need to, but I don't live and wallow in them any longer.

I have discovered that even in a disaster, enough remains to build on and to build from. Recovery has morphed into discovery, and my biggest regret now is that I didn't embark on this journey sooner. It's easy to say "I wish I had ..." but it's more joyful to say, "I can't wait to ..."

Knowing that with each breath comes the possibility to make a change and a difference is more comforting than focusing on what could have been. The realization that I got sober at just the right time to handle what has come in the last 20 months is more powerful than the regret of not handling the events of the past to my full potential. My actions and the lifestyle I embody say more than my words could ever say, but this lifestyle of sobriety will allow me to speak the exact truth at the perfect moment for someone who needs to hear it because they also want that lifestyle.

I began going to therapy about seven years ago for depression and suicidal ideation. But drinking clouded or washed away the truth I sought. I tried to take my life in 2016, and despite having consumed enough alcohol to register a .36 BAL at the hospital, along with about a month's worth of Xanax, my liver saved me once again. I woke up to a police officer, two paramedics, and my parents standing over me in tears.

Even after rehab and lots of therapy, I continued to slowly kill myself with the contents of a bottle. But in a doctor's office in August of 2021, something didn't just click, it snapped. I could feel the right lobe of my liver through my abdominal wall as my doctor told me to either stop or die. He said he would be there with me if I stopped, but he had to move on from me if I chose to drink one more time.

At that moment, I had reached my lifelong capacity for telling lies. I just couldn't tell one more lie. So, I embarked on a journey of freedom that came with each admission of guilt or deceit. Soon I realized that living in truth came easier because the results were predictable and cathartic. I didn't need to keep up with which lies I told to which person, and that freed my mind to find the truth within myself.

The truths I discovered about myself were difficult to face, but each one carried a valuable lesson. They helped me build a foundation upon which I could firmly stand, no matter what life brought. The pain I endured as a child and caused as an adult gave way to self-love and understanding. I realized that I had done the best I could, but that "best" was never what others needed, because alcohol never allowed me to see past my own issues and selfish needs.

Now, although the truth often sets me free, it doesn't do so until it has finished teaching its lessons. But now, when it declares, "Here endeth the lesson," I face new opportunities to grow. I no longer need to create drama to have a reason to drink. Now, I just show up and wait to see what is in store for me next. And I do so now with excitement and wonder in place of dread.

I look forward to sharing that experience with others to help them find their own paths of discovery. I look forward to the next sunrise, the next laugh with my children, and the next opportunity to grow and experience what things may come. But all the while I breathe in the now, and I am forever grateful for that.

ROXANNE E.

"My story is from the other side of addiction, as a daughter and wife, who has lived both in the disease and in recovery. I have never known a day in my life without either." A mother to three sons and one daughter and a grandmother to eight. I am a child of the 60's and in love with life. I am an innovative thought leader and activist. I have been in family recovery for 43 years, and for that, I am eternally grateful. My favorite go-to song is Patti LaBelle's, "People."

Growing up in the arena of active alcoholism is, for the most part, a traumatic, chaotic, and soul-numbing way to live. As the oldest of four, I learned to survive by becoming skilled at reading the room and by shapeshifting to whatever I needed to be in any given situation.

I learned to fake it till you make it by holding my breath and hoping it would soon go away. I learned to hover over my own life, living in the space of total denial. When I look back, I see that I paid a price, often not in that moment, but in the emotional, physical, and spiritual wounds caused by 18 years of living in the disease of addiction.

Yet, with all that said, I have also been blessed to have over 43 years of active recovery in my life. Loving and living with someone in recovery can be both terrifying and transforming. Both my father and husband are what I call my qualifiers. Each time they were in the throes of their addiction, I was called upon to find that space within me to show up from a place of courage, finding the compassion needed for both of us to come out on the other side.

With my father, it took time. I was not a fan of his early recovery. I was 24 when he took his last drink September 7, 1973. And as much as I was relieved that he was sober, the scars of my upbringing made this newfound happiness in sobriety seem like a cruel joke. I was angry and resentful and wanted nothing to do with either my dad or my mom. But then I believe my higher power intervened. Seven years into his recovery, my dad called and said, "How would you like to go to a woman-to-woman conference with your mother?"

I reluctantly said, "Sure." So, in September 1980, I flew to Brownsville, Texas and spent the weekend with 100 AA and Al-Anon women. For those three days, I learned that when two or more are gathered to share their experience, strength, and hope, miracles happen. There was a lot of laughter and hugs, tears, and sadness, and yes, at times anger, at a disease that robbed both sides of the aisle of their childhoods, marriages, careers, aspirations, and relationships—but most of all their dignity and peace of mind.

My miracle that weekend was that I heard their stories. I saw their transformation. I felt their sincere effort to show up differently. And most importantly, I saw myself in them.

I saw a scared young woman who was afraid to let go of the story of what this disease had done to her. I saw a woman who no longer knew how to set boundaries or be honest about the discomfort she lived with in her own mind, body, and soul. I saw a woman who had a wonderful life patiently waiting for her.

After that weekend, I started rebuilding a new relationship with my parents. I started going to meetings for Adult Children of Alcoholics, and other conferences, and slowly began to trust this new way of living,

And then in 1991, I fell in love with a friend I had known for

15 years. Dynamic and charming, he was skilled at spinning the story of, "I do not have a problem." But I had been around this disease too long to not understand the gaslighting and denial going on between us.

I called my dad one day and said, "Dad, I think I fell in love with one of you guys."

He laughed and said, "Of course you did."

My father helped my husband by sending him talks from other alcoholics in my husband's profession. On September 9 of that year, my husband took his last drink.

Again, as happy and relieved as I was that he had stopped drinking, I learned very quickly that there is a difference between being sober and being in recovery.

We who live with the alcoholic immediately heave a sigh of relief when they get sober. We begin to see positive changes and a newfound sense of stability. We have a glimmer of hope because, for many of us, recovery was not always a one-and-done. It was years of broken promises and gut-wrenching disappointments.

But as much as there is a relief that he was not using, this was new territory for both of us. Early in recovery there can be something called dry drunks. It's behavior that mimicked the drinking days, yet the person is sober.

That has always been one of the hardest things for me to deal with. My history of growing up in this disease caused me to get triggered if I sensed behavior that mimicked the drinking days. We were not married at the time he stopped drinking, so I had to trust that he was doing what he needed to do to work his own program, and I needed to continue to work mine.

Once we were married, my husband and I both realized we needed the help of those who had gone before us. They call them "old-timers," but their wisdom and the commitment to helping those early in sobriety saved our marriage and, in many ways, I believe they saved our lives.

We learned the importance of open and honest communication. Again, it was not always easy. We would go to meetings together—he to AA, me to Al-Anon. We had a couple's group that met once a month. We believed it was a family disease, therefore, it was a family recovery.

Our children began to hear a new language, see sayings on the chalkboard of "One day at a time," "Easy does it," "Progress, not perfection." And the serenity prayer now hung in our living room. We did not hide the recovery; we embraced it in all walks of our life. My husband and I learned how to trust again, to be gentle with each other through both our words and our actions.

We did a weekly check-in with each other, not to fix each other, but to really listen with an open heart. We would start by saying our name as we did in meetings. We each shared what was on our mind and heart. The only ground rule was the same as at a 12-step meeting—just listen, without judgment or comment. We then ended it with the serenity prayer. We did that every Sunday for 20 years. That last Sunday he said, "I am so grateful for the life I have been given with you and our family. I knew the path I was on before recovery would not end well."

I will be eternally grateful that my husband got his 28-year chip five days before he passed away suddenly on October 2, 2019.

One of the hardest things for me in my own recovery was to take the focus off the alcoholic. I was so practiced at reading the room, the mood, and the tone, that I had lost my own ability to take care of myself. I quickly learned by going to meetings and hearing others share their own experiences, strengths, and hopes, that I needed to start looking at my part in this dance of recovery. I was skilled at being their cheerleader and providing them with encouragement, but it was time I started doing that for myself.

I learned that being in a good marriage was not being with the perfect person, it was about me showing up every day and being the best partner I could be. The other day I heard someone say, "We were recovery partners." I smiled and thought, Yes, we were.

I have realized over the years when I go to meetings that it is not so much about what I share, as it is about what I hear. One time I heard, "I needed to give him the dignity to be wrong!" That statement has stayed with me for 40 years. By listening to other people's stories, I learned to take the focus off the addiction and allow those I love to walk their own journey.

It has been tougher with our kids. I could walk away from my father, I could walk away from my husband, but to walk away from a child is contrary to everything I knew.

One of the byproducts of growing up with addiction was that I became hypervigilant and always looked for the next shoe to drop. It was, and is, exhausting. So, I began to learn to be less judgmental; to allow them to share their own fears and perspectives and beliefs without pointing out they were mistaken or incorrect. I learned to engage in dialogue that promotes understanding and empathy, instead of attacking or belittling them for their thoughts or behavior.

One day when I was obsessing over one of my children, I heard my child's higher power say, "There is not room on the path for all three of us." I have never forgotten those words. And I learned that fixing them was never about them, it was always about me doing whatever it took to make it all go away. I still must be vigilant about not wanting to fix things. I can quickly go into that arena fully ready to do battle. However, it was not my battle to fight.

While it was important for me to understand the difference between the disease and the person, it was equally important for me to establish and maintain personal boundaries. I became more practiced at recognizing situations where I needed to respectfully disengage from discussions that had become disrespectful, hurtful, or unproductive. Sometimes I would forget that just because they were sober did not mean that the addictive behaviors would automatically stop. Just as I was practiced in my own unhealthy reactions, they were practiced in theirs. It took time, and I still periodically slip into old behavior. But now I quickly catch myself, smile, and tell myself I need to call a friend in the program or go to a meeting.

I have also learned that if I wanted my husband or kids to be vulnerable and show up in a new way, I had to let them know it was safe to do that by showing up from a place of empathy and compassion. I had to demonstrate what my mentor Brené Brown calls, Courage over Comfort. I had to learn to understand and to look at the underlying reasons rather than focus on their actions.

In doing so, I had to become vulnerable. I had to learn when I was triggered by their behavior to not react, but to respond in a way that helped us both. I learned to be curious and open to their reasoning. I would ask, "Can you help me understand?" instead of, "Why would you do that?" My favorite is, "The story I am telling myself." Many of us are so practiced at creating a story and then cherry-picking whatever we need to verify our story. I would find myself resentful, which was because my own expectations had not been met. I look back and realize how often I gave hours of energy and a good night's sleep to a situation I had created in my own mind, only to find nothing happened.

I believe that building the connections, both within recovery communities and with my loved ones affected by addiction, helped me become the person I am today. I strive to live a whole-hearted life, embracing my imperfections and practicing authenticity.

Step 9 of AA addresses our making amends to those we have harmed. It is not easy to absorb the reality and look through the eyes of rigorous honesty in how we who lived with this disease can also cause harm. My father was the first to teach me about "living amends." The best amends we can make is to become the best version of ourselves—to show up being a good human, making positive and consistent changes, and when given the chance, to pass it on.

Recovery has given me a pathway to live a meaningful life. I have been able to let go of my past, learn from my experiences, and show up as the best version of me. I can be the life partner, mother, grandmother, daughter, sister, friend, and the activist I wanted to be. I was able to have a 15-year friendship and a 28-year love affair with a man who met me every day on the field of recovery, put out his hand, and said, "Let's do this together!" And for that I am eternally grateful.

LOUISE ATHEY

Louise found herself in an AA meeting in March 2009, put down alcohol three weeks later, and through AA, therapy, the discovery of a higher power, and a lot of work, she has been sober ever since. Having taken a break in 2020 from a career in financial services to write a novel, she discovered that she might not be going back to her old career. While the novel is not yet published, she started working as a meeting leader for The Luckiest Club, offering sober mentoring. Now she spends her time helping others live a happier sober life. She has several projects going on—some writing, some healing—and she is much more open to a life of possibilities instead of a defined path. As well as her work in sobriety, travel, live music, friendship, and walks with coffee also fill her soul. She is now excited by the tomorrow that she used to dread.

Louise lives in the south of the UK with her two kid-adults and her black lab, Lola.

But …. and this is a big but … what if—hear me out—what if this might be the best decision you ever made? How would that be?

Sorry, I know. You said, this is the end; I hear you. I understand that you think your life is over. Sorry, you know, do not think. Your life is over, I heard you. Yes, you couldn't possibly be an alcoholic. Of course, I agree, ridiculous.

Absolutely. You don't drink all day, or every day. You don't need it to get up or go out. I agree, you don't need it, full stop. We don't need to debate that. The idea is shameful, of course. Yes, I know. Still ridiculous. Obviously, you're not homeless. Obviously, you have a job. Yes, I can see clean clothes. I know you ate.

Alcoholics live on park benches, are old men wearing dirty coats that are held together with string. Yes, I know. Although they weren't, were they? They were all very well dressed, some of them exceptionally so. In fact, it wasn't what I was expecting, not at all. And what's with the counting how long they've stopped for, what on earth is that all about? How can that be something to celebrate? Wouldn't you expect them to keep quiet about it? Accept the shame. And certainly not be laughing. How can they laugh when this is the end? I hear you. Laughter was way inappropriate.

Yes, I know. Not drinking alcohol is a crazy idea. I mean, who would do that? Apart from alcoholics, obviously, nobody. And, yes, it's not like you need it. It's just a drink, right. And of course, if you'd known that was what they were going to suggest, you wouldn't even have come. Evidently, I don't know how you eat spaghetti Bolognese without a glass of red wine or watch a rugby match without a pint of beer. And of course, your daughter will get married and there'll be champagne, I completely understand. But she is only six, so that is quite a way off. What sort of response is giving it up? It's just a case of getting hold of it. Sorting it out. Managing it. Controlling. I know.

You say it's part of being a grown up? Really, is that what you think? That it's a reward? Do you need a reward? Of course, I see. Validating. All appropriate.

Being an adult is difficult; I can't argue with that. But that doesn't mean you have to choose a reward that's damaging. Can't you find a different reward? Some kind of treat, maybe?

I'm sorry; I don't mean to be patronizing. I'm not belittling you, not at all. I'm trying to understand. I want to understand why you are doing this to yourself and why the suggestion of stopping is so impossible. Especially since you're telling me that you don't need it.

What's the worst thing that could happen if you did stop?

But, if you leave that to one side for a moment, what about just trying? How about stopping and seeing how it goes? Isn't that what they've all done—stopped? Could that be the answer? Or even a possible answer? Surely it's worth consideration. They seem so happy, so content in themselves. Are you listening to them at all?

What if you tried? Do you think you could stop? Sorry; I see I am repeating myself. Who stops anyway, of course. And why would they stop?

What about if you consider that problem drinking exists on a spectrum. That the alcoholic is at one end of it and that maybe you're yet to get to that.

That's still awful? Oh, right.

It's not like it hasn't always been a problem for you. It's not as if you ever drank safely. It's always felt like playing Russian roulette, never quite knowing where it's going to take you. I've always been worried about it for you. Don't you want that to end? Don't you want better and more? A life where that isn't always there, always at the back of your mind?

How much time does it take, do you think? Going back over the last disaster, replaying how it could have gone differently. Projecting into the next one, working out how it isn't going to be a disaster. Planning every move, every conversation, every non-drink.

Do you think people who can drink normally think about their drinking? Do you think they have a relationship with alcohol, or is it just a thing that they do.

You want to go and do some more drinking and then come back? You want to go and watch it, now that you know more. Do you think that will work? What if you can't come back? What if your drinking becomes so bad that you can't find your way back? What then? What if you do something so awful that you don't get a choice? What if you hurt somebody else? What about your children?

Don't look at me like that. What makes you think you're safe from doing something awful? Why should you be any different? You're thinking about stopping because it's a problem. Because you have no control. Because every so often you can't stop. What if, that one time that happens, you do that one thing too much. Can you write that drama, that story? Can you work out how you come back from that?

You want to start tomorrow? Won't that become the new thing, though? I mean, there's always going to be a tomorrow. Always.

Remember the times when you changed how you drank? What were they about? Only drinking at the weekend, only drinking at home, only drinking red wine or white wine. Only beer, only when you are out. What were you trying then? Trying to find a way that you could drink, trying to find the perfect pattern? What if you don't have a perfect pattern, what if you just can't? Can't. Maybe. You. Just. Can't.

You need to remember the mornings waking up when you didn't know where you were or how you'd gotten home or whom you were with. What about those? How would you feel if your children had those? What would you want for them? What is stopping you from wanting that for *you?*

Admit it. You can't stop. Admit that there have been times when you have wanted a drink when you woke up. Admit that you have wanted a lunchtime drink. Admit that you've lied about your drinking. Admit that you wish you could drink like a normal person. Admit that your drinking has gotten you into trouble at work and at home. Admit that you have lied—lied to yourself and to others. You have lied to the people you love. You have hidden it. You know that you have.

You need to stop lying to me; I have been through all of this with you. It's time you faced into the truth. Now, not tomorrow —today.

How can you live without it there beside you? What on earth do you mean? Celebrating your wins, commiserating your lows, is that what you think it's doing? It's not your best friend. Can't you see that? It doesn't want to hold your hand, it wants you lying dead in a gutter.

This won't be the end; it will be the beginning. Please, can you want this? Please, can you want a new beginning? Please find your-self worthy of more. Please.

Look at the people who have stopped. Look at what they're doing. Listen to what they're saying. Can you feel it? These people aren't at all what I was expecting. Although I don't know what I was expecting, did you? They seem happy, don't they? I mean, that is actually comforting.

Don't think about forever; try just thinking about today. I know, crazy, because obviously it all adds up to forever and, yet again, ridiculous. But let's just do now: this day, this hour, this moment. You're not drinking now. Can you do that, just that?

You think maybe you can? Maybe. I know, this can't go on like this; it needs to stop. I agree. You can do this. You can get to a better place, you will get to a better place.

So, I guess it starts here, then. No time like the present. Tomorrow will have to wait.

And who knows, this could be the best decision we ever make.

LISA MAY BENNETT

Author of *My Unfurling: Emerging from the Grip of Anxiety. Self-Doubt, and Drinking.* Sobriety and self-publishing are her passions.

After decades of drinking, I finally realized that alcohol was not my friend. When I was drunk, I often said and did stupid things and ignored my own health and safety. I usually felt awful the next day, and in the long term, drinking kept me from pursuing my dreams.

As I write this, I am six years sober and have very little desire to drink. Deciding to quit was one of the most amazing gifts I ever gave to myself. My life is much fuller. I like to try new things. I'm more adventurous. I wrote and self-published a book! I am mindful about my actions, more focused on my wellbeing, and careful not to engage in overblown arguments with loved ones (those were never pretty).

One of the keys to my success was breaking the link in my mind between common events and consuming alcohol. During those first couple of years, I had to struggle through: making dinner without a glass or two of wine; numerous birthday and anniversary celebrations where I was the only one not drinking;

and countless evenings when all I wanted to do was to unwind and forget my troubles.

I learned to sit patiently with the cravings that arise when I feel stressed out by work, home, and caregiving responsibilities. Now, I no longer "need" a drink at the end of a tough day or even a difficult week. But what about those times when the pressure has built for months? This is when I'd like to drink again, if only temporarily.

Vacations, long holidays, and even three-day weekend getaways are triggers that don't happen often, so they are more challenging to reprogram. We all need a chance to decompress, to set aside our worries for an extended period. The goal is to embrace a vacation state of mind as quickly as possible. And I learned early on that nothing speeds up the relaxation process quite like alcohol.

The last time my husband and I took a trip before I gave alcohol the boot, we flew to Florida to visit friends. I remember hurrying to our gate at the airport and plopping down at the closest bar. We ordered a beer and a margarita and texted our friends a photo of us clinking our glasses. That "cheers!" announced that we were free from the drudgery of everyday life. We were officially off the clock.

My husband and I haven't gone on an overnight trip in three years due to the pandemic and my mother's declining health. Recently, we were on a "staycation" with plans to do lots of outdoor activities. But due to bad weather, we mostly toured the food and beverage establishments in our area. A nice vacation, but not the one I had envisioned.

One evening, we were sitting in a local brewery after finishing a pizza from the food truck outside. As I sipped my bottled water and watched my husband drink his draft beer, I got antsy.

Most of the time I don't mind watching other people consume alcohol. People who drink enthusiastically, as I did, typically have spouses, friends, and family members who enjoy drinking. When I decided to get sober, I knew that those closest to me would not necessarily follow my lead. I've come to terms with that fact. My brain knows that drinking is a bad idea for me. But decades of conditioning deep inside still proclaims that "time off" is meant for drinking.

For many of us, a break means sleeping in, chillin' as much as possible, and drinking more than usual. Hey, we've earned the right to throw out the rulebook and do very little for the time we have. As someone who juggles a part-time job with a budding career as an author and the role of my mother's health advocate, I need to cut loose sometimes, too.

As I settle into my sobriety, I've started looking at vacations differently. I continue to believe that a break from my daily routine is good. I want my precious time off to seem special, out of the ordinary. But lately this has led to overindulging in sweets, and the result feels very much like an awful hangover.

So, I've made a promise to myself that I will use my vacation and holiday time to do activities I normally can't fit into my busy schedule. Yes, fancy meals are fun, and I will continue to accompany others to breweries, wineries, and distilleries. But I will also book memorable experiences for myself and whoever wants to join me. I've also started saving to go on a yoga retreat one day—my dream vacation.

If changing how you think about time off sounds interesting to you, too, here's a list of some of the new things I've tried over the past six years, plus a few things that are on my to-do list for future vacations:

Acupuncture (this can be very relaxing)

Aerial yoga (many of the physical activities on this list have introductory classes you can take)

Bungee fitness class

Cooking class

Dance class

Escape room

Flotation therapy

Hatchet throwing

Hiking

Indoor rock climbing

Kayaking
Massage
Meditation class
Paddleboarding
Painting or crafts class
Pilates
Pole or chair dance class
Qigong
Rail biking
Sauna
Sound therapy
Tai Chi
Topgolf
Trampoline Park
Zip-lining

PEGGI COONEY

Social Worker/Teacher/Coach/Writer/Former Blackout Artist and Cognitive Dissonance Expert living her sobriety out loud, so others don't have to. Author of *This Side of Alcohol.*

The Sober Social Worker: Lessons from Sara
By Peggi Cooney

I had been a child protective services social worker for less than a week when a sheriff's deputy asked me to meet him at an apartment complex in a small, rural town about twenty minutes from my office. This was my first call out. My first case. I was full of anxiety and self-doubt.

When I arrived, I observed two toddlers, close in age, wandering around the living room. They were drooling and crying. The shirtless tots were covered in dried milk, their leaking diapers so soiled and full of urine they nearly dragged on the floor. There was also a boy who looked to be about seven years of age sitting cross-legged on a chair. He looked down at the carpet and refused to make eye contact with me. Their mother Sara (not her real name) was face down, passed out on the couch, an empty handle of vodka beside her on the floor. The deputy had a difficult time waking her up.

How could a mother love vodka more than her beautiful children? I'd wondered at the time. Over the next few years working with Sara and her children, she would teach me just how wrong I had been.

It was no coincidence that Sara was my first child welfare case. She showed me that love had nothing to do with addiction. I learned that Sara fiercely loved her children, and they loved her right back. Sara wanted to stop drinking. She tried over and over again. At the time, AA was the only option, and she didn't feel comfortable attending because she didn't want the whole town to know her business.

I was overjoyed when Sara finally agreed to an in-patient program, and it was me who drove her to rehab and filled out her admission papers. Her hands shook so bad that she couldn't sign her name. (Little did I know that years later, I would be looking down at my own shaking hands.) Sara surprised everyone by completing the entire six-month program and proudly walking out of that facility after being alcohol-free for 183 days. We all thought she was on her way to a different life for herself and her children.

Sadly, it wasn't long before Sara went right back to drinking and eventually succumbed to her addiction—leaving three children without a mother. I still look back on her death and wonder what I could have done differently to change the outcome.

Fast forward about a decade. After sixteen years of being exposed to daily child and vulnerable adult abuse, I began to feel the effects of vicarious or Secondary Traumatic Stress (STS), which is defined as:

The effect of hearing and being impacted by emotionally disturbing and shocking experiences from clients. In hearing these traumatic experiences, child welfare workers go through an internal process of making sense of these experiences. Additionally, STS consists of a list of symptoms that are similar to those of PTSD, such as intrusion, avoidance and arousal.[1]

On top of STS, the system trauma I experienced was even

worse. Children would disclose they were abused, then find themselves forced to live with complete strangers in foster homes. It hurt my heart. It hurt my soul. On particularly stressful days, I began to pour myself a glass of wine after work to relax. I deserved it, right?

My friends and family justified those glasses of wine with comments like, "I don't know how you do it." "Your job must be so stressful." "I could never do what you do; it would break my heart." "Of course, you need something to take your mind off what you see every day."

When my drinking turned into a noticeable habit, people around me made it easier for me to continue. I call this secondary denial, where others unknowingly gave me permission to drink. My apologies for embarrassing or unforgivable behavior were followed with: "Peggi, you work so hard." "You weren't that bad; you just need to eat when you drink." "You were really funny last night." (Was I? I don't remember a thing.) "With your job, you deserve to relax."

"Don't worry, you're fine," they told me.

I wasn't fine.

A few years later, I retired from direct social work practice. Within fourteen days, I was hired by UC Davis to teach social work for the California Northern Training Academy. Teaching for the academy was and continues to be a dream job. Once out of direct practice, I was no longer experiencing the effects of vicarious trauma. I excelled in the position, and four years later received an outstanding service award for my work. But I remember thinking that if they really knew me, they wouldn't have given me the award. I drove home feeling like a complete fraud and proceeded to drink an entire bottle of wine alone.

It would take me another year and almost losing my family to admit I was addicted to an addictive substance. Another year of suffering the shame, utter self-hatred, and cognitive dissonance of teaching social workers how to work with families affected by addiction and then stopping by the store on the way home to buy a bottle of sauvignon blanc. Another year of comparing and rationalizing my drinking. A year of stepping in and out of AA meetings, telling myself, "I am not one of *those* people."

Surely, I could get this drinking thing under control.

But I couldn't.

During my last year of wine, I had increasing episodes of partial or full memory loss. I woke up almost daily with at least a low-grade hangover. I was full of "hangxiety." I denied and lied. I know that sometimes it was easier for my husband Paul to go along with my lies than to confront me because my reaction was often either volatile or hysterical. I made promises and broke them. Just like Sara.

I hadn't planned for July 11, 2019, to be my last drink. We had rented a cabin in Lake Tahoe for an annual family picnic. My daughter, her husband, and their two sets of twins—ages three and six at the time—walked in on Paul screaming at me because I was drunk. The next morning, she said, "Mom, if you do not do something about your drinking, you cannot have the relationship you want with me, Jason, and the kids."

The price was finally too high to pay. I could not have hated myself more on that day. I went into the bedroom, got down on my knees and heard these words, "Peggi, you are done, and you are going to be okay." I signed up for the Sober Sis 21 Day reset within an hour. Thank God, after at least a hundred attempts, I was finally done. I have been alcohol-free for close to three-and-a-half years now.

In so many ways, I am grateful I had a drinking problem. I am a completely different person in recovery. I am confident and present. I am learning to let go of the past. I discovered that I am a writer. There is no denying that I am a better human, wife, mother, grandmother, and friend. I am the teacher that my social work students deserve to have, which positively impacts the children, families, and adults they work with. I can gently (and sometimes not so gently) lead students to a more compassionate and trauma-informed practice. I work for a university that encourages me to live my sobriety out loud—something many first responders are unable to do.

Rest in peace, my dear Sara. You taught me so much. Know that I will take it from here.

thissideofalcohol.com

Facebook.com/groups/thissideofalcohol

@thisisideofalcohol

---

1. Hatton, H., Brooks, S., & Borucki, J. (2014). *Associations Between Health, Workplace Support, and Secondary Traumatic Stress Among Public Child Welfare Workers: A Practice Brief.* Northern California Training Academy, University of California, Davis.

GERALDINE BLOOMFIELD

Sobriety has brought light, clarity, compassion, and truth, to bring her home to herself. She can generally be found in a yoga pose, the sea, or a conundrum. She is grateful for sober connection, love, family, nature, freedom and her beautiful friends, many of whom are in TLC. Geraldine is from Sussex in England and is a research communications specialist.

A message to my day-one self:
"Warning: Geraldine, there is a hostage situation. I repeat, a hostage situation. You are being held by a captor whom you mistakenly think you love and cannot escape from. You are in grave danger. Geraldine, this is your soul talking. Do you copy?

Your toxic imprisoner has controlled and preyed on your family for generations.

There is a way out. But you must listen to me. I repeat, you must listen to me. Do you copy? Over."

This persistent, quiet, fervent SOS was coming from deep inside, alerting you to danger, Geraldine.

You were living in a Stockholm syndrome situation.

Stockholm syndrome is a clever and devastating psychological coping mechanism that occurs when someone is rendered powerless, trapped, and held against their will. Bizarrely, the prisoner appears to be in collusion.

It is essentially a paradoxical mind trick that we play on ourselves to endure abusive and terrifying times. At its core, it's a survival tactic—a bewildering and brilliant one.

And you knew it well, sweet day-one Geraldine.

Now, two years into recovery from alcohol dependency, you can see the truth of your constriction. You can understand the warped, befuddled trickery that was at play. Back then, you didn't see it. No clue. Ziltch. Nada. No frigging idea.

When freedom came knocking with a release, a moment of escape finally showed itself. A rock bottom of the soul propelled you toward a higher, better life.

Geraldine, on your day one—a desperate, dreary Sunday back in January 2021—you absolutely did not comprehend the danger you'd been in. You couldn't yet see how alcohol had held you confined, sick, and small.

Alcohol had you against your true will. It kept you shrouded in a protective fog of denial. You were gaslit by the myth of booze as necessary, enjoyable, and essential. Cheered on by family, by friends, by society, and yes, by your own pickled mind.

Deep inside of you dwelled a quiet but tenacious voice who knew the truth. But she was almost impossible to hear from within the prison walls.

Your jailer kept you ill and unaware.

And you liked it. You needed it. You relished your time with it. Alcohol supported you. Enlivened you. You panicked when it was gone. You pined for it. Craved it. You *had* to have it. It was your first thought upon waking: *Did it visit last night? How nice was it? How bad did it make me feel? Will I see it again today?*

My advice, dear day-one broken self, is to understand the super-toxic soup of Stockholm syndrome that you were swimming in.

Alcohol has been your warden, not your savior.

You had convinced yourself that you were in love because you were afraid to drown in the painful truth. Even at the point of breaking free, you don't quite see that it is the nightly wine and weekend gins that make you anxious, depressed, and uninspired.

You'd been enslaved by the insidious, enchanting hold of alcohol. And you are not alone. Many live there too.

You believed you had no choice. You were stuck—no decision, agency, or free will. You did not question it.

But don't feel bad or ashamed. This is bossy, brutal alcohol doing its job.

Luckily for you, you have a rebellious streak. An obstinate, determined part of your spirit which refuses to remain silent or obedient. She is your light, your potential, your divine creative force bestowed by the cosmos. She is a freedom fighter. And she was on a mission to give you a different, bigger, bolder, brighter life outside the gates. Away from that too-small space in which you were crammed.

When your soul could bear the pain no more, she burst in, Navy SEAL-style, to perform the life-saving rescue mission you never realized you needed.

And how could you? In a sense, you'd grown up in the dark, musty, heady cell of addiction. From the first drink at 13, you'd been bound. You hadn't known there was another way.

After all, alcohol drips from the branches of your family tree: the always-drunk uncles, the abusive and hard-drinking grandfather, the party-time parents. These characters were the norm in the story of you.

At 11 years old, you wrote a personal narrative about you as a toddler. It was meant to be a "funny" anecdote for your teacher about how your 18-months-old self would mosey around your family's Sunday gatherings to steal and sip from finished beer bottles left out in the afternoon sun. There are pictures to prove it.

"Oh, starting early," the adults would remark.

"One of us," they'd laugh.

Through no fault of their own, your parents gave you a beer-bottle shaped identity which entrapped you.

As psychiatrist and addiction expert Gabor Maté says, addiction is the quest to access the true authentic self. Alcohol use gives you momentary, tantalizing glimpses of that self. And with it, the relief. Yet, it's not your true higher self. It's still the false self, masquerading. At first this feels divine. Something pure. But it is the illusionary fog of liquor. It is a lie. A trap.

You thought you could not function alone. That you could not come down from your working week without the reward of a Friday night blow out. That you could not celebrate a birthday, enjoy a holiday, attend a wedding, lose a loved one, misplace a purse, or even fill in a form alone.

Your controller, alcohol, told you that you'd be unable to travel without him; that you'd be unable to host a party, attend a work trip, have lunch with your mother, or take the kids camping without him. He was convincing. And full of bull.

When your soul radioed the truth and gave you the spark of awareness, you picked up your tools to start your escape. You began running toward the horizon, away from that bully.

At times you were fearful that he was gaining, ready to snap at your feet and ensnare you once more.

But now you've found your pack, your people, all on the same path. You can slow a little now, knowing that you've crossed the sober border into a new land. You are safe. You are no longer in survival mode.

Your true life was waiting. That life is steeped now in abundance and wonder, rife with the promise of content mornings, fruitful afternoons, meaningful connections, and playful creativity. A peaceful, wide-open life without the clanking of prison keys.

You walk with pace and purpose. And when you cannot, you rest and give yourself the repose and replenishment you need. You have direction and desire, a gentle commitment to healing. You have an inner love.

You understand, though, that you still don't call the shots. Your abuser is no longer in charge, but something else greater is. It reigns with compassion and love, not fear and shame. It has awakened you to the big mystery of the universe, and it grants you, when you pay attention to the signs, the life you need.

Today, the soft wisdom of your heart has unlocked your life. She shows you peace. She shows you joy. Serenity, even.

So, dear reader, hold your ear to your own heart, can you hear a soul SOS? A faint yet distinct—*dot, dot, dot; dash, dash, dash; dot, dot, dot*—tapping below all the fervor, all the noise?

That, my friend, is your spirit, signaling for escape from the confines--quietly, urgently screaming for freedom.

For the release of the undeniably more real, more true, more beautiful you.

ALIX ALDERMAN

Boy mama, fascinated by spirituality, science and nature, redwoods, raptors, oceans, night skies. Biopharma innovation executive. Former perfectionist and gymnast. Recovery is rebellion, freedom from conditioning.

What didn't you know about the brain and body effects of alcohol?
By Alix Alderman

I first fell deeply in love with science as a young girl, enraptured by its potential to unravel the intertwined complexities of our world and arm us with knowledge to help us understand, innovate, and thrive. I was awe-struck by the vastness and smallness of the world all at once—the starlit night, the massive redwoods, a tiny intricate shell with a soft life inside. I followed this innate curiosity and passion toward a scientific degree and then embarked on a 20-year career researching and developing new medicines for rare genetic diseases. I've witnessed the power of science to completely transform lives.

All that scientific knowledge was useless, however, when I

found myself in the tight grip of alcoholism. For years, I'd used willpower as my lone armament in a draining, repetitious psychological battle against this powerful beast. I relied on medical facts, logic, duty, fear, and shame to motivate and berate myself into resisting the unrelenting urges to drink. I tried desperately to catch a breath, as the pace of life accelerated on a wild treadmill that threatened to throw me off at any moment. There was no rest from combat as this brain disease progressed, no respite from my fear of defeat.

Paradoxically, the sole action required to sever the chains of addiction and gain freedom from this cognitive prison is to raise the white flag of surrender.

Only when I learned to let go of control and lean into connection did the constant clamor in my head quiet. Being held in a safe net of community with fellow travelers and seekers restored my nervous system and brought forth an invitation to know myself with compassionate curiosity. The audacity to sit in stillness with the nature of my mind steadily widened my aperture to consciousness. With increasing awareness, agency and practice, suffering and fear gave way to freedom and connection. I came home to my true self, and with that homecoming came a deep sense of belonging and purpose.

During my drinking years, I thought I was well aware of the effects and consequences of alcohol, such as liver problems and regrettable decisions, but there was so much more I did not know. I have come to learn that ethanol takes an incredibly serious toll on our overall mental and physical health through acute hijacking of biochemical feedback loops, followed by long-term rewiring and reinforcement of disruptive brain circuitry. *Stress—a physiological response when demands on our system, mental or physical, exceed our coping mechanisms—has everything to do with addiction.*

In an attempt to maintain homeostasis when under attack by stress, our brain and body discharge chemicals and release hormones. In chief is cortisol—"the stress hormone"—which is key to understanding and intervening in the addiction cycle. What starts as insidious damage to our nervous system and organs through alcohol-induced cortisol flooding becomes entirely pervasive, both soul-crushing and life-threatening over time. Even moderate chronic drinking can trigger widespread cortisol-potentiated inflammation and affect virtually every organ and tissue throughout our body, including in our heart, brain, lungs, eyes, skin, gut, and immune system. Alcohol is a carcinogen and a literal poison, determined by the World Health Organization to be a toxic substance with no level of consumption safe for our health.

Learning about the fascinating science of addiction and neuroplasticity, which is the brain's ability to reorganize and develop new neural connections, transformed everything about my recovery. I came to understand that in the depths of my drinking, I rode a wild stress paddlewheel, bathed in alcohol and cortisol that literally changed my neural circuitry. Cortisol disrupts the architecture of our sleep and leads to interrupted and low-quality sleep, specifically less of the REM sleep during which our body and brain heal and recharge. As a result, we operate on an increasingly empty tank with wounded infrastructure. Ethanol disrupts our gut biome by killing the healthy gut bacteria that support feedback between our digestive system and brain, a communication loop that is vital toward normal central nervous system functioning. This disruption of the gut biome and nerve cell activity has been implicated as a factor influencing mental illnesses, including depression and anxiety symptoms.

As most people in recovery discover, many entangled layers lie beneath the outward manifestation of addiction behavior. We create our brain over time by the inputs that we receive—those from our own mind and body and those from our external environment, relationships, and the nature of our nurturing.

My compulsive thinking started long before my compulsive drinking. I was a great test case for the power of recovery to change the brain, as I was hard-wired for habit by early conditioning toward perfectionism and self-reliance. I spent over 15 years of my childhood as a dedicated gymnast, embedded in a culture of verbal, physical, and psychological abuse. We gymnasts were meticulously corrected and viciously berated for small mistakes. We learned to work tirelessly for praise and perfection, rewarded by hard sought but fleeting moments of complimentary attention. The conditioning began early—the push to stand out, to achieve, to get the mark, the medal, the praise, the win, the thing.

We were taught by threat of shaming to hide our feelings, to push through fear, physical and emotional pain signals, and to never share with our parents about what happened in the gym. I learned to not speak of my suffering; instead, I diligently managed everything in my own head, relying on hypervigilance and fear-based planning.

When I began to squarely look at where my fears and internal chaos originated, it was edifying to discover much of this was embedded in my inner voice. The berating, brutal way I talked to myself had taken on the same tone of my gymnastics coaches: "You're an idiot." "You're being lazy." "Work harder." "Stop it." "Get it together." These daily narrations continued long after I had retired from gymnastics and well before my drinking progressed.

Where our attention goes, neural connections grow. Connections become pathways, and with increased use, these well-trodden circuits form automated habits. After years of fear-based motivation to achieve success and please others, I became hard-wired for rumination—a stress-based, personal narrative all centered around fear of failure. These persistent, intrusive thoughts ultimately carved deep pathways of anxiety, depression, and craving. Many of us drink simply to quiet rumination, welcoming the prison break, a respite from the enslaving bonds of our burdening thought loops.

The process of recovery is one of truly reclaiming who we are and our freedom to choose where we place our attention. I had very little freedom when I was drinking; I grasped onto thoughts, I attached to craving. Fortunately, we can recover our true essence and our health; we can recalibrate our internal equilibrium and natural balance with the world. I could only regain freedom by summoning the willingness to crack my armor, by letting my fearful self be carried by a recovery group as I progressively opened wounds and worked to heal them.

Despite my pupa state, my community infused sufficient courage for me to try the experiment of surviving without the only medicine I knew. Taking alcohol out of the equation forced me to feel the intense discomfort and to look at how my own thinking and resistance had driven my suffering. But in that pain, I found more opportunities to ask for help—and in turn, more connection.

It was suggested that I speak to myself as I would to my young son, if he were suffering: "You're okay." "You're in the right place." "This will change." "I'm here to help you through this." "You are not alone." I developed patience with myself and reframed the internal voice that I used.

Much like the young girl I once was, I now start each day and close each night with gratitude and acknowledgement of the beauty, wonder and awe in the world. These actions place my attention and energy outside of myself and connect me spiritually with something bigger.

Over time, the compounding toll of ethanol and cortisol had translated in ebbing glow, a pallor across my skin, eyes, and psyche. When I finally put down the alcohol for good, the vibrant light returned to my irises, an outward manifestation of the renewal and burgeoning connections within.

The lens with which I view the world, and how all of life unfolds, has completely shifted. I have slowed down, and I value stillness and grounding as portals to guide me where to place my attention and action next, which is essential to my purpose and service to the world. As a result, I feel far more connected and present with my son and loved ones, more creative, more productive, and more accomplished in my work.

My husband, who was diagnosed with a devastating episodic disease that takes him away from us for periods, suffers often in pain with no cure. But I now can pivot into service when he is sick, without the rest of life crumbling. I can ask for help. I can support my son as he navigates the unknown, the big feelings and experiences of childhood.

I can be confused, make mistakes, fall down, get back up and grow as we humans are intended. I can offer calm and solutions when there is chaos at work, when egos clash, or when financial stress hits. I can show up for difficult and necessary conversations, knowing how to persuasively and kindly influence change without shrouding in fear. I no longer fight with myself or with the world. My head has become a peaceful place to live.

I've discovered that intention, attention, spirituality, and my connection with the universe and energy all around us, have literally changed my brain. For me, the brain changes necessary for these practices, harnessing this inner power, could only have come with first putting down the drink. I am forever grateful for the always-present guides who are there for each of us on this journey, every step of the way, if we seek them.

We are never alone, and we can all transform. We simply have to want it, to reach out, to practice, and hitch ourselves to the universe. The flow and balance that returns to our own primatial ecosystem in turn restores our flow and balance with the infinitely more massively complex interdependent ecosystems, and the results of our inner work ripple outward into everyone and everything, ad infinitum.

INSTAGRAM RESOURCES

Sober, Sober Curious & Healing Spaces on Instagram	Instagram	Mission
Alex Elle	@alex_elle	Essayist; Writing Coach; Joy Seeker – Internationally Healing
Anne Lamott	@annelamott	Writer
Brene Brown	@BreneBrown	Storyteller and Research on the power of vulnerability
David Whyte	@davidjwhyte	Poet and Philosopher
Discover Earth	@discoverearth	Stories to bring you hope from around the globe
Dry Together	@drytogether	For women age 35-60 around the world who are redefining the role of alcohol in their lives
Emily Paulson	@emilylynnpaulson	Founder of @sobernumsquad and author of Hey, Hun and Highlight Real
Finding Mastery	@findingmastery	Taking you inside the minds of the best in the world
Gabby Bernstein	@gabbybernstein	Author. "New Thought Leader." Oprah
Glennon Doyle	@glennondoyle	Author; podcast host of "We Can Do Hard Things."
Cory Allen	@HeyCoryAllen	" I write slow thoughts for fast times".
Holly Whitaker	@holly	Author: *Quit Like Women*
Professor Andrew Huberman	@hubermanlab	Neuro Scientist, Stanford University

Jolene Park	@jolene_park	Gray Area Drinking expert
Know Thyself	@Knowthyself	A place to discover more about the true nature of self
Kristi Coulter	@kristiccoulter	Author: *Exit Interview: The Life & Death of my Ambitious Career*
Laura McKowen	@laura_mckowen	Author: *We are the Luckiest*; *Push Off from Here* Founder of The Luckiest Club – a global sobriety support community
Loosid, Live Sober, Love Sober	@Loosidapp	A Sober Social Network
Maureen Anderson	@maureen.j.anderson	Sobriety Coach & Mentor
Megan Wilcox	@sobahsistahs	Alcohol-Free Life Coach
Mel Robbins	@melrobbins	Author, Researcher, Podcaster @themelrobbinspodcast
Melissa Urban	@melissau	Whole 30 Founder & Author: *The Book of Boundaries*
Deb Podlogar	@Mocktail.mom	Sharing non-alcoholic drinks & the fun of sober living
Nedra Glover Tawwab	@nedratawwab	Author; Therapist; Relationship & Boundaries Expert
New fashioned sobriety	@newfashionedsobriety	Alcohol-free community based in WI, USA
Dr Nicole LePera	@theholisticpyschologist	Psychologist; Author: *Do the Work; How to Meet Yourself*
On Being	@onbeing	Wisdom to replenish and orient Podcast
Pandemic Sober Squad	@pandemicsobersquad	The PSS supported, and continues to do so, those getting and staying sober during the pandemic with loving kindness and a wicked sense of humour
Peloton Sober Strong Squad	@pelotonsoberstrongsquad	A group of Peloton members who are in Recovery, Sober, Alcohol Free or Sober Curious

Recovery is the New Black	@recoveryisthenewblack	Normalizing sobriety in our boozy culture. Keynote speaker & Author: *Living Sober, Living Free*
Trina Turner	@theRetiredPartyGirl	Sober mother. Supporting women to up-level their lives through self-discovery
Sam Harris	@Samharrisorg	Neuroscientist, philosopher and author. Host of the *Making Sense* podcast and the creator of the *Waking Up* app
Sans Bar	@sans_bar	Virtual Academy for sober bars and bottle shops
Scott Barry Kaufman	@Scottbarrykaufman	Cognitive Scientist. Founder of the Centre for Human Potential
Sober Girl Society	@sobergirlsociety	Sober Girl Society | Community for sober + sober curious women
Sober Motivation	@SoberMotivation	Sober Motivation
Sober Powered	@sober.powered	Quit drinking with good science. Podcaster.
The Luckiest Club hosts:		
This Side of Alcohol	@ThisSideofAlcohol	Author; Speaker; Social Worker; Trainer; Coach & AF advocate sharing thoughts of pain, hope, humor, love and all that is possible in sobriety
The Sober Millennial	@the_sober_millennial	Digital creator doing sober things; doing gay things
The Nap Ministry	@Thenapministry	Examining the liberating power of naps. We believe rest is a form of resistance & reparations. REST IS RESISTANCE!

Amanda E. White	@Therapy For Women	Retired Party Girl → Realistic Therapist. Host: Recovered-ish Podcast
Thich Nhat Hanh	@Thichnhathanh	Zen Buddhist monk, peace activist and author. This account is supported by monastic and lay Dharma teachers in the Thich Nhat Hanh tradition
Annie Grace	@ThisNakedMind	Health & wellness website. Change Your relationship with alcohol (and have fun doing it)
Umbrella Dry Drinks	@umbrelladrydrinks	Non-alcoholic bottle boutique + bar
Vex King	@vexking	Author: Closer to Love: How to Attract the Right Relationships and Deepen Your Connections Co-founder @therisingcircle Kindness | Positivity | Evolution
We the Urban	@wetheurban	Celebrating self-love, inclusivity, & marginalized voices
James McCrae	@wordsarevibrations	Planting seeds for a better world. Author. Teacher. Meme Poet Founder: @sunflower.club.creative
Becky Vollmer	@YouAreNotStuck	Writer, teacher, speaker, dreamer Yoga, empowerment, sobriety Author: *"YOU ARE NOT STUCK"* Host of THE CIRCLE
Yung Pueblo	@yung_pueblo	Meditator. Author: The Way Forward Co-Founder @wisdomventures
Susie	@Zeroproofexperiences	Validates a Zeroproof Lifestyle. Sober in the City, Traveling Event
Sober Movement	@sobermovement	Promoting sobriety as a lifestyle
The Sober Grind	@sobergrind	One (Funny) Day at a Time

Sober Curious Collective	@sobercuriouscollective	Celebrating life beyond alcohol. Come on an adventure with us
The Sober Glow	@thesoberglow	Musings from a teetotaling, silver-haired broad
Sober Butterfly Collective	@soberbutterflycollective	Spread your wings & fly into a #sober social life
Sober Vibes	@sobervibes	A community for #Sober and #Sobercurious women
Virtual Hope	@Virtual._.hope	An interactive learning platform

RECOMMENDED READING

We are the Luckiest: The Surprising Magic of a Sober Life
Laura McKowen

Push Off from Here: Nine Essential Truths to Get You Through Sobriety (and Everything Else)
Laura McKowen

Drink: The Intimate Relationship Between Women and Alcohol
Ann Dowsett Johnston

Drinking: A Love Story
Caroline Knapp

Big Blue Book: Alcoholics Anonymous
Alcoholics Anonymous World Services

Quit Like a Woman: The Radical Choice to Not Drink in a Culture Obsessed with Alcohol
Holly Whitaker

Untamed: Stop Pleasing, Start Living
Glennon Doyle

The Easy Way to Control Alcohol
Allan Carr

This Naked Mind: Transform your life and empower yourself to drink less or even quit alcohol with this practical how to guide rooted in science to boost your wellbeing
Annie Grace

The Alcohol Experiment: How to take control of your drinking and enjoy being sober for good
Annie Grace

Dry : A Memoir
Augusten Burroughs

Blackout: Remembering the Things I Drank to Forget
Sarah Hepola

Between Breaths: A Memoir of Panic and Addiction
Elizabeth Vargas

Sober Curious: The Blissful Sleep, Greater Focus, Limitless Presence, and Deep Connection Awaiting Us All on the Other Side of Alcohol
Ruby Warrington

Nothing Good Can Come from This: Essays
Kristi Coulter

The Recovering: Intoxication and its Aftermath
Leslie Jamison

The Book of Awakening
Mark Nepo

When Things Fall Apart: Heart Advice for Difficult Times
Pema Chodron

Start Where You Are: A Guide to Compassionate Living
Pema Chodron

Girl Walks Out of a Bar: A Memoir
Lisa F. Smith

Love Warrior
Glennon Doyle

Twenty Four Hours A Day
Alcoholics Anonymous

You Are Not Stuck: How Soul-Guided Choices Transform Fear Into Freedom
Becky Vollmer

Sober Lush: A Hedonist's Guide to Living a Decadent, Adventurous, Soulful Life— Alcohol Free
Amanda Eyre Ward

The Sober Diaries: How One Woman Stopped Drinking and Started Living
Clare Pooley

The Unexpected Joy of Being Sober: Discovering a Happy, Healthy, Wealthy Alcohol-Free Life
Catherine Gray

Sunshine Warm Sober: The unexpected of joy of being sober—forever
Catherine Gray

The Sober Girl Society Handbook: An Empowering Guide to Living Hangover Free
Millie Gooch

Sober on a Drunk Planet: Giving Up Alcohol. The Unexpected Shortcut to Finding Happiness, Health and Financial Freedom
Sean Alexander

Being Sober: A Step-by-Step Guide to Getting to, Getting Through, and Living in Recovery
Harry Haroutunia

Dopamine Nation: Finding Balance in the Age of Indulgence
Dr. Anna Lembke

Confess
Rob Halford

Cold Turkey: How to Quit Drinking by Not Drinking
Mishka Shubaly

I'll Push You: A Journey of 500 Miles, Two Best Friends, and One Wheelchair
Patrick Gray, Justin Skeesuck

I Swear I'll Make It Up to You: A Life on the Low Road
Mishka Shubaly

Atlas of the Heart: Mapping Meaningful Connection and the Language of Human Experience
Brené Brown

Brené Brown Collection: Daring Greatly, Dare to Lead, Rising Strong
Brené Brown

Living Sober
Alcoholics Anonymous World Services

Twelve Steps
Alcoholics Anonymous World Services

Twelve Traditions
Alcoholics Anonymous World Services

Tiny Beautiful Things: Advice on Love and Life from Dear Sugar
Cheryl Strayed

In the Realm of Hungry Ghosts: Close Encounters with Addiction
Gabor Maté

Parched: A Memoir
Heather King

Tired of Thinking About Drinking: Take My 100-Day Sober Challenge
Belle Robinson

The Spirituality of Imperfection: Storytelling and the Search for Meaning
Ernest Kurtz & Katherine Ketcham

Lit: A Memoir
Mary Karr

Healing the Fragmented Selves of Trauma Survivors: Overcoming Internal Self-Alienation
Janina Fisher

Man's Search for Meaning
Viktor Frankl

The Untethered Soul: The Journey Beyond Yourself
Michael Singer

The Gifts of Imperfection
Brené Brown

WOLFPACK: How to Come Together, Unleash Our Power and Change the Game
Abby Wambach

The Awakened Brain: The Psychology of Spirituality and Our Search for Meaning
Lisa Miller

The Comfort Crisis: Embrace Discomfort to Reclaim Your Wild, Happy, Healthy Self
Michael Easter

*Ten Percent Happier: How I Tamed the Voice in My Head, Reduced Stress Without
Losing My Edge, and Found Self-Help That Actually Works—A True Story*
Dan Harris

Self-Compassion: The Proven Power of Being Kind to Yourself
Kristin Neff

Recovery: Freedom from Our Addictions
Russell Brand

My Fair Junkie: A Memoir of Getting Dirty and Staying Clean
Amy Dresner

Broken: My Story of Addiction and Redemption
William Cope Moyers

Clarity and Connection
Yung Pueblo

Lighter: Let Go of the Past, Connect with the Present, and Expand the Future
Yung Pueblo

Inward
Yung Pueblo

What Happened to You?: Conversations on Trauma, Resilience, and Healing
Oprah & Dr. Bruce Perry

Emotional Sobriety: From Relationship Trauma to Resilience and Balance
Tian Dayton

Let's Take the Long Way Home: A Memoir of Friendship
Gail Caldwell

The Biology of Desire: why addiction is not a disease (The Addicted Brain)
Marc Lewis

The Liars Club
Mary Karr

The Leadership Challenge: How to Make Extraordinary Things Happen in Organizations
James M. Kouzes

Recovering from Emotionally Immature Parents: Practical Tools to Establish Boundaries and Reclaim Your Emotional Autonomy
Lindsay C Gibson

I'm Just Happy to Be Here: A Memoir of Renegade Mothering
Janelle Hanchett

Mother Hunger: How Adult Daughters Can Understand and Heal from Lost Nurturance, Protection, and Guidance
Kelly McDaniel

The Road Less Travelled: A New Psychology of Love, Traditional Values and Spiritual Growth
M. Scott Peck

One Day at a Time
Al-Anon Family Groups

Courage to Change: One Day at a Time
Al-Anon Family Groups

It Works: How and Why
Narcotics Anonymous Fellowship

The Path to Recovery: A Guide to the 12 Steps
Chasity Bailey

Breathing Under Water: Spirituality And The Twelve Steps
Richard Rohr

Relationships in Recovery: Repairing Damage and Building Healthy Connections While Overcoming Addiction
Kelly E. Green

The Gifts of Imperfection: Let Go of Who You Think You're Supposed to Be and Embrace Who You Are
Brené Brown

Exceptional: Build Your Personal Highlight Reel and Unlock Your Potential
Daniel M. Cable

This Side of Alcohol
Peggi Cooney

Face Yourself. Look Within
Adrian Michael

Emotional Sobriety: From Relationship Trauma to Resilience and Balance
Tian Dayton

I Didn't Believe it Either: My Discovery That Everything Is Better Without Alcohol
    (Available Dec. 2023 on Amazon and ToddKinney.com)
Todd Kinney

Love Wins; Everything is Spiritual
Rob Bell

A SAMPLING OF QUOTES FROM OUR AUTHORS THAT HAVE HELPED THEM

Wherever you go, there you are. –Alen Watts

When we remember we are all mad, the mysteries disappear, and life stands explained. –Mark Twain

One day at a time.

This is the singular, hard truth I come up against every day: I am the only one responsible for my experience. –Laura McKowen

Feelings come and go like clouds in a windy sky. Conscious breathing is my anchor. –Thich Nhat Hanh

I want to believe that the imperfections are nothing—that the light is everything. – Mary Oliver

It is never too late to become the person you were always meant to be. –George Eliot

Rest in the mess. –Unknown

Be with life and myself as it is, and as I am. –Unknown

The typical question is, "Is this bad enough for me to have to change?" The question we should be asking is, "Is this good enough for me to stay the same?" And the real question underneath it all is, "Am I free?" –Laura McKowen

We only fail when we stop trying. –Unknown

Our deepest fear is not that we are inadequate. Our deepest fear is that we are powerful beyond measure. It is our light, not our darkness that most frightens us. –Marianne Williamson

You never have to get sober again –David M.

The struggle is real, so are the rewards –Jeff Graham

The serenity prayer

It's hard to get enough of something that almost works. –Dr. Vincent Felitti

Start each day with a grateful heart. –Unknown

Create a life you don't have to escape from. This quote really turned things around for me. It reminds me that I am in control of my circumstances and my life. I AM empowered to live a full, beautiful life, no matter what I have done or gone through in my past. –Holly Whitaker

Your opinion of me is none of my business. –Unknown

Live, travel, adventure, bless, and don't be sorry –Jack Kerouac

The opposite of addiction is not sobriety—it's connection. –Johann Hari

I care for myself by accepting others' care for me. –Sophie Araque-Liu

I have not come this far to have come only this far –Unknown

Shame, guilt, community, grace, hope, resilience. –My journey in 6 words.

Nothing will improve by taking a drink today. –Anonymous

If you get sober, you give yourself a raise. –Anonymous

Meeting Makers Make It. –Anonymous

Every Day Sober is a Gift. –Anonymous

It is not your fault. It is your responsibility. –Laura McKowen

If there's a book that you want to read, but it hasn't been written yet, then you must write it. –Toni Morrison

Don't ask what the world needs. Ask what makes you come alive and go do it. Because what the world needs is people who have come alive. –Howard Thurman

You are loved.

This, too, shall pass –Buddhist Mantra

What You Seek is Seeking You. –Rumi

Tell me, what is it you plan to do with your one wild and precious life? –Mary Oliver

I am superior to negative thoughts and low actions. –Anonymous

Choosing G.O.D. (Grace Over Drama)

We all have limited time, and we don't know how much of it. The difference between happiness and suffering or wisdom and confusion is using attention in a profound way; having the space to put your attention where you want it. You are really only as free as your attention is free to be put to good use. –Sam Harris

Progress over perfections.

There is no passion to be found playing small—in settling for a life that is less than the one you are capable of living. –Nelson Mandela

Don't question the decision. –Unknown

It's hard getting what you want from something that almost works. –Gabor Matte

Courage, dear heart. –A whisper from Aslan to Lucy in a book by CS Lewis

Love, Connection and Acceptance are your birthright. To claim them, you need only look within yourself. –Kristin Neff

Where the attention goes, the energy follows. –Unknown

Doing is work; Being is effortless. –Unknown

We all have choices; we just have to be brave enough to make them. The opposite of fear is choice. Change begins when we realize the life, we want doesn't line up with the life we're living after that, it's all about getting off autopilot. Intention without action is just wishful thinking. –Becky Vollmer

Push off from here. –Laura McKowen

Set your life on fire. Seek those who fan your flames. –Rumi

ABC. Always Be Curious. –Unknown

When I cannot bear outer pressures anymore, I begin to put order in my belongings...as if unable to control my life, I seek to exert this on the world of objects. It's as if outer order creates inner calm. –Anaiis Nin

There can be no happiness if the things we believe in are different from the things we do. –Freya Stark

You can't be true to yourself and play small at the same time. –Jodi White

Transformation doesn't ask that you stop being you. It demands that you find a way back to the authenticity and strength that's already inside of you. You only have to bloom. –Cheryl Strayed

Owning our story can be hard but not nearly as difficult as spending our lives running from it. Embracing our vulnerabilities is risky but not nearly as dangerous as giving up on love and belonging and joy—the experiences that make us the most vulnerable. Only when we are brave enough to explore the darkness will we discover the infinite power of our light. –Brené Brown

Choose your hard. –Brené Brown

Integrity is choosing courage over comfort; choosing what is right over what is fun, fast, or easy; and choosing to practice our values rather than simply professing them. –Brené Brown

Hope is invented every day. –James Baldwin

I drink. I just drink differently, and I deserve a pretty glass and a place at the table. – Susie Streelman/Zero Proof Experiences/Sober in the City

What else could be true? –Eric Johnson in TLC Meetings

The opposite of addiction is connection. –Johann Hari

Our deepest fear is not that we are inadequate. Our deepest fear is that we are powerful beyond measure. It is our light, not our darkness that most frightens us. We ask ourselves, 'Who am I to be brilliant, gorgeous, talented, fabulous?' Actually, who are you not to be? You are a child of God. You're playing small does not serve the world. There is nothing enlightened about shrinking so that other people won't feel insecure around you. We are all meant to shine, as children do. We were born to make manifest the glory of God that is within us. It's not just in some of us; it's in everyone. And as we let our own light shine, we unconsciously give other people permission to do the same. As we are liberated from our own fear, our presence automatically liberates others. –Marianne Williamson

Abstinence alone is not Recovery. –Unknown

Be curious, not judgmental. –Walt Whitman

Our deepest fear is not that we are inadequate. Our deepest fear is that we are powerful beyond measure...By shining our light, we liberate others to do the same. –Marianne Williamson

One day or day #1. –Unknown

Vulnerability is our most accurate measurement of courage –Brené Brown

Everywhere is the same place when you're drinking it's where the drinking is. –Luke O'Neil

Tell me, what is it you plan to do with your one wild and precious life? –Mary Oliver

He who has a why to live for, can bear almost any how –Viktor Frankl

When you're overwhelmed, place a hand on your heart & say: "There is still more right with me than wrong with me. This will pass. I'll get through this. –Cory Muscara

RECOMMENDED PODCASTS

- This Naked Mind with Annie Grace
- Unlocking Us with Brene Brown
- On Being with Krista Tippett
- Home podcast with Laura McKowen and Holly Whitaker
- Tell Me Something True with Laura McKowen
- Heart of the Matter with Elizabeth Vargas
- Ground and Gratitude with Lorilee Rager
- The Hello Someday podcast for sober curious women with Casey McGuire Davidson
- We Can Do Hard Things with Glennon Doyle
- A Sober Girls Guide podcast
- The Start Today podcast with Rachel Hollis
- The Mel Robbins podcast
- Soberful the podcast with Veronica Valli and Chip Somers
- Sober Gratitudes by Sarah Elizabeth
- Knockin' Doorz Down
- Adam Carolla Show
- The Bubble Hour with Jean McCarthy
- The One You Feed
- That Sober Guy Podcast with Shane Ramer
- Rehab Confidential with Joe Schrank and Amy Dresner
- Recovery Elevator with Paul Churchill
- Recovery Rocks
- Seltzer Squad-Staying Sober in the City
- Practice You with Elena Brower
- Armchair Expert with Dax Shepard
- Finding Mastery with Dr. Michael Gervais
- Huberman Lab
- Making Sense with Sam Harris
- The Sober Mom Life podcast with Suzanne
- Ten Percent Happier with Dan Harris

- Back from Broken - Colorado public radio
- Take a break from drinking with Rachel Hart
- Daily Reflection Podcast with Michael L. and Lee M.
- Dear Gabby Podcast: become the happiest person you know with Gabby Bernstein
- Tara Brach
- Recovery Happy Hour with Tricia Lewis
- Everything Happens with Kate Bowler
- SoberCast: An (unofficial) Alcoholics Anonymous podcast
- 1000 days sober podcast with Lee Davy
- OYNB (One Year No Beer) podcast
- The Unruffled podcast with Sondra Primeaux and Tammi Salas
- On Purpose with Jay Shetty
- The Chase Jarvis LIVE Show with Chase Jarvis
- The School of Greatness with Lewis Howes
- Making it Happen with Henry Ammar
- The Robcast by Rob Bell
- Editing our drinking and our lives with Jolene Park and Donnelley Rowley

PROGRAMS AND GROUPS

We recommend community and connection, regardless of where you find it. We don't promote any one specific program or group. This is just a list; we recommend you do what is best for you. Look at them all. Stick to the ones that fit.

- TLC (The Luckiest Club) - online meetings, loads of subgroups, encourages growth instead of dogma - and anything that resonates for you
- AA, but do whatever keeps you sober and mentally well enough to stay sober and grow
- Refuge Recovery
- Recovery Dharma
- Sonder Recovery (queer-focused)
- Get a therapist
- She Recovers
- CoDA (Co-dependents anonymous)
- Recovery 2.0
- SMART Recovery
- Brentwood recovery home
- Y12SR, friend support
- Lionrock—on-line home-based recovery with a curriculum
- Tired of Thinking About Drinking Fellowship programs
- I Am Sober app
- Reframe app & community
- Sober Buddy app & community
- RewYre_U
- This Side of Alcohol
- Sober In the City
- Soberful
- Hola Sober
- Recovery Elevator for online help
- This Naked Mind
- Sobertown

- Local Yoga studios
- Annie Grace's 30 Day Alcohol Experiment
- Sober Mom Squad
- Chicago AF
- Al-Anon
- Bac2Zero
- Joining book clubs
- SoberSis
- The Phoenix
- Ben's friend Hope

ACKNOWLEDGMENTS

Writing a book is harder than I thought and more rewarding than I could have ever imagined. None of this would have been possible without my friends that said "YES" to this book. Thank you, to each of you, from the bottom of my heart. Your vulnerability, honesty, and strength have been foundational to my sobriety, and I'm honored to share your stories with the world. The world is a better place thanks to people like you who want to help and inspire others.

I'm eternally grateful to Lisa May Bennett, who my friend (and author) Peggi Cooney introduced me to. Thank you for taking this amateur author through the self-publishing process and answering all my questions. Your guidance, suggestions and motivation propelled me to get this book done in 2023.

My life has had many ups and downs; thank you to my parents and sisters who have always been in my life through every chapter.

Thank you to Jeanette Littleton who edited this book, Get Covers for designing the cover, and the formatter/proofreader, R.W. Harrison.

Thank you to my friend and fellow sober mom, Jennifer Bridgman. Thank you for your editing contributions, advice and positive "keep going" energy you gave me throughout the process.

It's an honor to be mom to Landon, Layla, Parker, and Paxton. Thank you for asking me how the book was coming along, with your impromptu, nonchalant check-ins, which motivated me to keep going and get this project done. I hope you each know I'm your biggest fan, just as you are.

To my friends, you know who you are and I hope you know

how much I love and appreciate each of you. My life is better with you in it and I look forward to making many more happy memories with you.

Thank you, Laura McKowen, for writing *We are the Luckiest*. This book and TLC changed my life and I'll be eternally grateful.

More information about Vanessa can be found at www.Vanessa-McDonald.com

Made in the USA
Las Vegas, NV
28 December 2023

83616854R00194